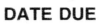
DATE DUE

rom Gothenburg,
ull time on issues
ly teaches sex edu-
ation to midwives,
as been appointed
ers regarding the
olence, and other
advisory council
.

PRINTED IN U.S.A.

RESPECT

Everything a
Guy Needs to
Know About
Sex, Love,
and Consent

INTI CHAVEZ PEREZ

Translation by Stuart Tudball

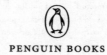

PENGUIN BOOKS

PENGUIN BOOKS

An imprint of Penguin Random House LLC
penguinrandomhouse.com

First published in Swedish as *Respekt: en sexbok för killar* by
Alfabeta Bokförlag AB, Stockholm

ISBN 9780143134251 (paperback)
ISBN 9780525506027 (ebook)

Printed in the United States of America
1 3 5 7 9 10 8 6 4 2

Set in Minion Pro
Designed by Cassandra Garruzzo

All names and identifying characteristics have been changed
to protect the privacy of the individuals involved.

CONTENTS

Going out

Talk to each other
Everyone argues sometimes
You don't own each other

Sex is not a must
Be equal together
The emotions roller coaster

Breaking up

Let your feelings out
Don't want to hurt anyone

Make the best of it

4. RESPECT

Show Respect

Guys in a Group

Respect technique #1:
Respect yourself

Groping

Respect technique #2:
Don't cross other people's boundaries

Sluttiness

Respect technique #3:
Stop spreading sexual rumors

Honor

Respect technique #4:
Don't control other people

Space

Respect technique #5:
Listen and give space

Talk about sex

Getting stuck in a rut

10. FEELING GOOD 185

Emotions

Shame and guilt
Going against your gut

Being forced into sex
Someone to talk to

Safer sex

Make a decision
How STIs work
Ways to make sex safer

HIV and chlamydia
Practice makes perfect
Get tested for infections

Pregnancy

Abortion
Contraception

Responsibility

THANKS

I would like to thank the people who read and commented on the book before it went to print:

Sandra Dahlén,
Mina Gäredal,
Johanna Hedlund,
Hilda Jacobsson,
Baris Kayhan,
Moa Keskikangas
and Luis Lineo.

Thank you to everyone who is quoted in the book. Almost all the names have been changed. Thanks also to RFSU, RFSL UNGDOM, and RFSL.

And finally, thank you Patrick Nolan, Matthew Klise, and the rest of the team at Penguin Books for making this book possible.

FIRST AND MOST IMPORTANT

I sometimes teach sex ed in schools. When I do, guys often want to know how to make sex feel good for both people. My answer is that respect is the basis for good sex and good love. A respectful union makes the sex on both partners' terms—and both get to enjoy it.

How that is done practically you'll learn later on in the book.

This book is aimed primarily at teenage boys. Your teenage years are a long time when a lot is going on. That's why I'm writing to guys who have never kissed anyone and to those who have already had a fair amount of sex. If something feels too advanced, just skip ahead and save it for later.

Good luck with love, and with sex.

—Inti

RESPECT

1

YOU

BELOW THE BELT

"Is my dick normal?"

"Is my dick normal?" is the most common question guys ask when they go to the youth clinic. They look at their penis and compare it with the others in the locker room. Then they worry that maybe theirs looks odd. And they're right; every penis looks odd because no two are exactly the same.

In most cases, guys are relieved to find out that their penis is perfectly OK. If you're concerned about your penis, you can go to the youth clinic and get checked out by a professional. But right now we're going to have an initial run-through of what a normal penis may look like.

Dick check

Pull down your shorts and we'll go through the different parts of the genitals, starting with the penis. If you're not circumcised, you'll have a foreskin covering the glans (head), but the amount of foreskin varies. In some guys the foreskin goes beyond the tip to form what looks like a trunk. Others have a shorter foreskin, so you can see the tip of the glans. The length of the foreskin makes no difference in any regard.

Some guys have a tight foreskin that hurts if drawn back. In such an instance it is worth having a doctor examine you. Sometimes a tight foreskin is due to age—you just have some growing left to do. In other cases, the foreskin may need a bit of help in the form of a special cream, for example.

Think about something that turns you on. This causes blood to flow down, making the penis grow in width and length; it gets harder, rises up, and gets warmer. It may also become redder.

If you hold your erect penis in your fist, you can feel that it's harder on the top, the side nearest your stomach. The underside and the glans are softer. The urethra runs through these parts, which have to be softer so the tube doesn't get squeezed. You can feel with your fingers that the erection continues all the way into the perineum, the area between the testicles and anus.

When you look at your erection, you'll notice that it is curved and off at an angle. The thickness is also uneven. No penis is entirely straight or regular, not even when soft. In the past, men's trousers used to be tailored to the lean. The tailor would ask which way the gentleman "dressed," whether the penis hung to the left or the right, and would adjust the trousers accordingly.

On the edge of the glans, by the urethra and the frenulum (banjo string), you might see little bumps that may be white. Over half of guys have these. The bumps tend to appear in puberty and are called penile papules. Some guys are concerned when they find these and think they have some sexually transmitted disease or pimples, but the papules are entirely harmless and cannot be removed with medication or soap.

Odd skin

If you ate a burger and fries every day, fat would collect in the body and it would make your thighs fatter, for example, but your penis wouldn't get thicker, because there is no fat layer under the skin of your dick.

The absence of fatty tissue makes it easier to see things under the skin of the penis. Veins show more clearly. There may also be bumps that stand out. These bumps are either hair follicles or sebaceous glands that lubricate the skin.

The penis has more pigment than many other parts of the body, so it may also be slightly darker. The pigment can be unevenly distributed and make the penis look splotchy.

On the penis there is a kind of ribbon that runs all the way from the banjo string at the top, down along the penis and perineum, ending at the anus. This ribbon can vary in its appearance and is almost invisible on certain guys. The ribbon is what's left of a seam that joined together the genital area when you were in the womb.

> If the banjo string on the glans is short, it can break and start to bleed. It can look pretty scary, but it isn't dangerous. See a doctor if this happens to you.

The scrotum moves

If you stand up, you'll see that one testicle is slightly larger and hangs a little lower than the other. Having them hanging at different heights allows you to move about without your testicles rubbing or knocking against each other. Imagine two bulls butting heads at full speed. That's what your testicles *won't* do!

The scrotum makes sure the testicles are at the right temperature to produce sperm. If you're wrapped up warm, your testicles will hang down. If cold air blows over the scrotum, it will shrink.

When you were in the womb, your testicles each sat in a separate pocket inside the body. Sometimes a testicle can creep back up into one of those pockets. It can be a little painful, as there's not much room in the pocket, but after a while the testicle will descend again. If you feel by your testicles with your fingers, you may notice something with the consistency of spaghetti. This is the epididymis, where the sperm grow to maturity and are stored until they leave the body.

Mix of fluids

When you masturbate, sooner or later a clear white fluid will drip from the urethra. This fluid is called precum, and its job is to clean out the urethra. The amount can vary significantly from person to person and time to time. Sometimes the precum only appears just before you come, but at other times you may see precum as soon as you get hard.

As you continue to masturbate, the pleasure gets greater and greater until you can't hold out any longer and you have an orgasm, where a wonderful feeling of pleasurable release washes over you. You'll generally ejaculate at the point of orgasm, although this may not always be the case. The muscles tense and the semen sprays out in spurts. The amount of semen ejaculated is usually equivalent to one or two teaspoons, but it varies and there may be more if you're going for a long time before you come.

The semen is a mix of fluids that come from different parts of the body. The actual sperm, the little tadpoles that swim around, are just a few hundredths of what makes up the semen.

> The sperm that reach the egg first don't fertilize it. What happens is that the sperm surround the egg and help each other to open it up. Then one of them can swim in and merge with the egg.

A guy once told me that he usually had white semen, but that once when he had sex, his semen was transparent like water. It only happened that one time. Then the semen went back to its milky color. This happened because the mix of fluids that make up the semen can vary from time to time. That variation is nothing to worry about.

Shortly after ejaculating, you may find that you need to pee. This is a bodily reflex to get you to flush out any remaining semen from the urethra.

The P-spot

One of the main ingredients in semen is a fluid made in the prostate gland. This substance can solidify and form clumps if you ejaculate in a bath, for example. The sperm would not survive very long in a girl's vagina without the substance, which is why the prostate is important for guys who want to be fathers. However, the prostate is also a sensitive part of the body that is sometimes known as the P-spot. Guys can be brought to orgasm by stimulating this spot, for example, with their fingers.

The prostate is about the size of a walnut. You can't see it, but you can feel it. If you insert a finger into the rectum, you'll feel a round bump about an inch in.

Exercise: Explore your body

For this exercise you will need one large mirror and one smaller, portable mirror.

Angle the portable mirror toward the large one so you can get a 360-degree view of your body. What do you look like from different angles?

Where do you have hair, birthmarks, or stretch marks on your skin? How does your erection bend when you look from the side?

If you press on your prostate gland, it can feel amazing, but at the same time you may feel like you need to pee, because the prostate in turn presses on the bladder.

When I was giving a talk in a school once, one guy shouted out "*Ewww!*" when I talked about the prostate.

"What's wrong with the prostate?" I asked. He answered:

"That's gay; don't talk about it!"

"But every guy has a prostate. If you think the prostate is gay, you must think all guys are gay?" I replied.

Because the prostate is reached anally, some guys find it embarrassing. But if you get to know your prostate and understand how it works, it can become a very enjoyable part of the body.

Erection for no reason

At some point, everyone has had an erection at the wrong moment. Maybe when giving a talk or wearing swimming trunks. Erections are simply something you can't control, and they aren't necessarily related to sexual arousal. The brain decides when you have an erection and can order one just to check that it works. If you want to get rid of an erection quickly, don't think about the erection itself. Think about something else that is sad or difficult, like war or the answer to 99 times 12.

You can automatically get an erection if something touches your penis—for example, if you're sitting on a train and your penis vibrates against your trousers or your leg. A full bladder in the morning can give you an erection as it presses against the nerves that control erections.

Buy cheap Viagra! Every day I see ads for pills to make my erection harder. But young guys don't need Viagra. Medicine sold online can be bad for your health. If you really think there is something wrong with your erection, see a doctor or nurse for help.

A friend recently asked me: "I sometimes notice that my boyfriend has an erection in his sleep. Is that because he's dreaming he's having sex or what?"

I explained that at certain times during sleep, you relax in a way that opens a flap and allows blood to flow down into the erectile tissue in the penis, and this causes an erection. It has nothing to do with sex dreams.

"Good, because I don't want him dreaming about anyone except me," said my friend, with a laugh.

Another common misconception about erections is that if a guy who likes girls eats contraceptive pills containing the female sex hormone estrogen, he will have an erection for several days in a row. Guys already have small amounts of estrogen in their body without taking contraceptive pills, so these pills would definitely not have any effect on erections. And you shouldn't take medicine that wasn't prescribed to you because you don't know what other effects it might have.

How to keep yourself clean

If you have a foreskin, you may have noticed that it produces a kind of oil that lubricates the glans. The oil is there to protect the glans, which is sensitive and doesn't like being touched by dry things.

If you're circumcised, the glans has a more leathery skin, which means it's not as sensitive and can manage without the oil. As the lubricant builds up, it becomes a sticky white substance known as *smegma*, or "dick cheese." So it's a good idea to wash inside your foreskin. When washing, make sure your foreskin is pulled all the way back. Use warm water but no soap, because soap dries out the skin, which can lead to an itchy fungal infection called jock itch. The penis has a natural smell of its own, which you shouldn't try to wash away.

Dick = dude?

Being born with a dick doesn't necessarily mean that you feel like a guy. You might feel that you're a girl or that you don't have a gender. This is called being transgender.

I have heard adults saying that "trans is a trend." They couldn't be more wrong. A person can feel utterly invisible when others constantly treat them as if they were a different gender. They might be given this book, for example, even though they don't think of themselves as a guy.

For the sake of a person's health, it's important that family, teachers, and friends accept the gender identity of the transgender person. They can do this by saying the right name and using he, she, or they correctly.

No one, not even a trans person, knows everything about themselves from the start. You discover who you are by testing things out. Trying different names, pronouns (he, she, they), and clothing allows you to find out what feels right to you.

APPEARANCE

Have you ever stood in front of a mirror, twisting and turning and tensing your abs and then thinking, *this does not look good*? Do you change your shirt, work some pomade into your hair, and then decide that it all still looks hopeless?

Everyone has been there. Even the coolest and best-looking guy you can think of has stood in front of the mirror and sighed about the things he thinks are wrong. A lot of the way you think about your appearance is determined by your own self-esteem, how confident you are, and how able you are to like yourself. If you're unhappy with yourself or with things in your life, you can also become unhappy with your appearance, no matter what you look like.

I'm not suggesting you'll suddenly get rid of all your zits and have perfect hair just because you have good self-esteem. You'll look exactly the same. What will change is the way you see yourself.

You shouldn't judge yourself too harshly. You might spend a lot of time finding fault with yourself in the mirror, but others tend to be a lot less critical of you than you are of yourself. What you see as bad or embarrassing flaws may well be things that other people don't even think about or care about—or may even find attractive!

Model and superhero

Films are full of guys you can compare yourself with, since most films have a male lead. But although there are so many guys on film, they're all quite similar. The lead male actor is mostly muscular, tall, and able to save children from burning buildings and disarm a bomb using a paper clip and some chewing gum. How great does that make you feel by comparison?

Comparing yourself with guys on TV or in ads is pointless. Their job is to be good-looking. They have personal trainers and stylists, they always wear makeup, they've sometimes had plastic surgery, and often both their appearance and voice are digitally enhanced. That's not something a regular guy can compete with!

Only half of young people between the ages of sixteen and twenty-nine are happy with their appearance and their body. This percentage is a sign that we compare ourselves with images we can't live up to.*

Personally, I think it's sad when people feel everyone should act the same and look the same. Everyone is unique, and that's a valuable fact that should be embraced. When you've discovered your true identity and how you want to live your unique life, you begin to like yourself, and that makes others attracted to you for who you are.

Good-looking enough for sex

Now I'm going to tell you something I thought was embarrassing a few years ago, but today I think it really doesn't matter.

Toward the end of junior high school, I had acne like everyone else, only worse. I had spots on my back that left scars, little dark marks all over the place. My acne scars felt a bit like a secret that I hid under my T-shirt. I never wanted to show off my upper body, and I was worried about sex. When I had sex, how would my partner react if my back was covered in dark spots? Would my appearance be good enough for sex?

*Source: The Swedish Agency for Youth and Civil Society, *Unga Med Attityd 2007* [*Young with Attitude 2007*] (Stockhom: The Swedish Agency for Youth and Civil Society, 2007), 46–47.

Since then I have had sex. And I've realized that sex is not at all how I thought. Sex is not particularly attractive; you're often breathless and sweaty. Sex is not about looking sexy or showing off your muscles. Sex is two people coming together, two bodies getting to know each other. And zits, bad hair, spindly arms, or spotty backs are actually irrelevant.

DICK SIZE

Anyone who has set foot in a men's locker room knows that guys are often obsessed with size. And it's not just confined to thirteen-year-olds. Interest in big dicks never seems to go away. When I was eighteen, some of my friends were surprised I didn't know exactly how many inches I had.

"You mean you haven't measured it!" they exclaimed, and ran to get a ruler for me. The largest penises I've seen have been in hetero porn, which is porn for guys who like girls. It seems that many guys find large dicks fascinating to look at. In our culture, a large penis is a symbol of masculinity and sexuality.

Too much importance is attached to the role of the penis in sex, and so many people think the bigger the dick, the better the sex. But good sex is by no means all about the penis.

Too small for intercourse?

"But what if I stick my dick into a girl and she doesn't even feel it?" asked one guy once.

"That's very unlikely," I answered.

Even if your erect penis is the size of a pinky finger, that's still something anyone will feel in their vagina or rectum. No penis is too small to be felt. Also, the first few inches of the vagina are some of the most sensitive. Farther in, the vagina loses its sensitivity, which means it doesn't matter if your penis is very short.

And yet many guys still worry about size. This is because a lot of people have the wrong picture about how sex works. They think there's a hole, and you have to fill that hole. But that's not how it is.

Both the vagina and the sphincter muscle in the anus are tight when a person is not horny. In this state, sliding a finger in would hurt the person. However, the vagina and the sphincter muscle expand when the person is aroused and you can warm things up with your fingers. Only then will the penis fit in.

Both the vagina and the sphincter can be expanded even more. After all, a baby can be pushed out of the vagina! You could say, then, that the vagina and the anal sphincter adapt to the situation—so a dick can't be too small for sex.

Exact inches

Many guys want to know exactly how big a penis others have so they can compare themselves. Personally, I think such comparisons are pointless because the size doesn't affect the sex. But because I'm asked so often to share the statistics, here they come.

A study I read shows that the average length of an erect penis is around 5 inches. The study was conducted on adult men, so you shouldn't compare yourself with this figure if you're still a teenager.

> You shouldn't believe guys when they tell you how big
> their dick is. Studies show that when asked about the
> size of their penis, guys tend to exaggerate by a few inches
> compared with the figure researchers get when they
> take out the tape measure.

The differences in penis size are greatest in the soft state, for example when comparing with others in the locker room. The differences occur because penises empty different amounts of blood as the erection goes away. The difference in size between two penises is therefore less in an erect state.

Pills and operations

When I read various online forums about sex, I sometimes come across posts from guys asking whether there is anything they can do to make their penis bigger. My answer to that question is no; at least there is no safe and effective way.

The pills advertised online are certainly not worth trying. Think about it. If they really worked, wouldn't they be advertised on TV so more people could buy them? There are no pills that make the penis grow. In the worst case, you might get something dangerous if you order these pills from the internet, and in the best case what you'll get are vitamins . . . just ridiculously expensive ones.

There are also devices available online that are supposed to stretch out the penis. These do not make the penis longer and can damage the erectile tissue that fills with blood when you get an erection.

Surgical procedures are also not particularly good. Operations commonly lead to damage and can even lead to impotency. With length operations, the few extra inches tend to quickly get eaten up as the cuts heal.

The only safe, long-term solution for those who are concerned about their penis size is to become more confident in themselves as people: to believe that you can be loved and give pleasure to other people. In that way, you'll be happy with yourself as you are and never give a second thought to the size of your dick.

FEELING HORNY

Johan is eighteen and in his senior year of high school. When we talk about feeling horny, he says, "I've never been as horny as when I was in junior high. I'm still very horny, but back then I was like a rabbit, going round being horny all the time."

He describes his horniness as something that occasionally got in the way of the rest of his life.

"It wasn't exactly easy to solve math equations when I felt like that. At times, the horniness took over completely, and all I could think about was quickly finding a bathroom so I could relieve the pressure. I know it was the same for my friends. We talked a lot about feeling horny, and although we didn't discuss jerking off in the bathroom, I think the others also did it."

And it wasn't without its problems.

"Sometimes it felt like being so horny was sick. Like when I'd jerked off four times and it hurt, but I just had to do it again. I thought there was something wrong with me," says Johan.

Don't be ashamed

The reason why teenagers feel especially horny is that the body is awash with hormones at this time of life. The hormones have a wide range of effects. The skeleton grows, the testicles begin to produce sperm, and the voice changes as you hit puberty. You also start to feel hornier.

Even if you think that being horny is a problem, it's a bad idea to try and suppress it. If you happen to get an erection when you're in public, or when you don't mean to, that's a different story; if you just remain calm and think nonsexual thoughts, it should eventually go away. But suppressing your emotions is never a good thing.

> Our sexuality is often with us from childhood. Half of boys discover masturbation before they reach their teens, and many have played sexual games with other children at a young age.*

I once heard a radio interview with men from religious families. As teenagers, they'd heard that feeling horny was bad. They weren't

*Source: Shere Hite, *The Hite Report on Male Sexuality* (New York: Knopf, 1981), 1093–94.

allowed to masturbate or fantasize about sex or they would end up going to hell, and so they tried to bury their emotions in every way possible. But of course they couldn't, and so their mental health began to suffer. One guy even convinced himself that he was a sex addict, despite not even masturbating!

If you ever feel that being horny is a problem, try to ride it out rather than putting up resistance. Jerk off when you feel like it, and remember that you're hardly alone in being super horny.

Not being horny

"The image of guys is that we're always horny and people joke about us thinking about sex all the time. But what happens when you don't want any sex? It's as if you become less of a man," says Ali, who is a few years older than Johan.

Ali recognizes himself in Johan's story. He has been extremely horny and enjoyed a lot of sex. But there are times when Ali doesn't feel horny at all and has no interest in sex.

"I like sex, but that doesn't mean I always want it. Sometimes I can go a month or more without wanting it. This doesn't mean sex has stopped being enjoyable, just that I don't feel the desire for it," says Ali.

He feels the picture generally painted is that if a guy isn't horny, there must be something wrong with him. Either he is ill or he has stopped being in love or he is even cheating.

But there is nothing wrong with not feeling horny, just as there is nothing wrong with you if, now and then, you don't fancy listening to music or you'd rather be alone than meet up with your friends.

SOLO SEX

Masturbation is having sex with yourself, and it is much simpler than having sex with someone else. With masturbation, you're the only person who has to want it, and you decide what happens. It's a good way to find out what you enjoy and to learn how to touch a person in a way that feels good.

Many people have jerked off since they were children. Others come to masturbation later. Karl began masturbating when he was ten or eleven.

"It was at summer camp and an older boy told us about a thing you can do with your hands. I didn't really understand what he meant, but when I tried it later it felt good," says Karl.

According to Karl, the hard thing about jerking off is that he lives with his family and has to hide it. He has his own room and has always been able to have time to himself, but when he hit puberty, semen began appearing and he had to go to the bathroom to get rid of it. Now he always has a roll of toilet paper and his own trash bin in his room.

"I empty the bin myself so mom doesn't see how much toilet paper is in there. My parents see it as a sign that I've begun taking more responsibility for cleaning my room and they're pleased," says Karl with a laugh.

No side effects

Guys have sometimes asked me whether masturbating can have any harmful effects. They think jerking off is a little too good to be true.

And it's not surprising to question it, as history is littered with all sorts of strange ideas about masturbation. *Onanism*, for example, is another word for jerking off that actually comes from a man in the Bible named Onan who was killed by God because he wanted to have sex without having children. That's enough to worry anybody!

> "The boy after a time becomes weak and nervous and shy, he gets headaches and probably palpitations of the heart, and if he still carries it too far he very often goes out of his mind and becomes an idiot."*

The most common question I've encountered is whether the quality of the sperm gets worse if you masturbate. Maybe you're wasting sperm and then you might find it hard to have children later on? The truth is that you continue producing sperm all your life, whether you masturbate or not. Your body is also not interested in keeping old sperm. If you don't masturbate or have sex, the body will eventually get rid of the sperm while you sleep. When this happens you might wake in the morning and notice you have damp underwear.

Another thing guys sometimes wonder about is why their penis can hurt after masturbating or having sex. This is also nothing to worry about. It's because the nerves in the penis have had a good time

*Source: Robert Baden-Powell, "Continence" from *Scouting for Boys: The Original 1908 Edition* (Oxford: Oxford University Press, 2005), 351.

and need to rest. If you just leave it alone for a while, the pain will go away by itself. However, it's not harmful to jerk off again if you want.

Some ways to jerk off

Guys are sensitive in different places and have different flexibility. Everyone's body is different, and so we also masturbate in different ways. Some ways may be more common than others, but that doesn't mean there's anything wrong with finding your own way of pleasuring yourself. Here are a few examples of what you can do.

HAND

Wrap your whole hand around your penis. If you have a foreskin, pull it back and forward over the glans. If you're circumcised, you can do the same movement, but it might feel more pleasurable if you squeeze some lube into the palm of your hand. If you don't have any lube, saliva can work, but it dries quicker.

RING

Touch your forefinger to your thumb to form a ring. Place the ring around the root of the penis and squeeze until it feels good. Move the ring up and down.

SELF-SUCK

Some guys can suck themselves off, usually if they have a large penis or are very flexible. Some can sit up and suck, while others need to lie on their back and bring their genitals up and over toward their head. Warning! If it's not working, don't push it. You don't want to break your neck.

How men usually masturbate*

82 percent use their hand to stroke their penis

24 percent stroke themselves all over their body

18 percent stroke their scrotum and testicles

15 percent rub themselves against their mattress

14 percent conduct anal play

7 percent play with their nipples

1 percent don't masturbate

0.5 percent suck themselves off

RUBBING

Lie on your stomach on the bed or on a pillow and rub your penis backward and forward. But remember that precum and semen can leave stains!

CONDOM

Roll a condom onto your penis. Masturbate with your hand or rub yourself against the bed. When you come, you don't need to worry about stains as the semen will collect in the condom. Later in the book, you can read about how to put on a condom correctly.

STROKING

Lightly touch your body with just the back of your hand, your fingertips or a feather. Stroke your face, lips, arms, chest, stomach, thighs,

---

*Source: Hite, *The Hite Report on Male Sexuality*, 1106.

and butt. Everyone likes different things. Do you have any parts of the body that you particularly like touching? Warm up the rest of your body before you do anything with your penis.

COMING

Have you watched porn and wondered what it feels like to get cum on you? Try it for yourself. The easiest way is just to lie on the bed and come on your stomach and chest. But if you lift your ass by placing a pillow under it or leaning up against a wall, you can also come on your face and in your mouth.

SOAPING UP

Make sure you have a damp body and wet hands. Use liquid soap and stroke yourself. Let your hands glide over your penis and maybe let a finger slip through the hole in your ass. This is actually best done with lube and no water. Lubricants are sold at the pharmacy.

SALIVA

Spread saliva over your penis. Let a fingertip glide back and forth over your penis and scrotum. Close your eyes and imagine it's someone licking you!

FINGER

Stroke your ass for a while first and relax. Make sure you don't have long or sharp nails. If you want, you can roll a condom over your finger to feel clean. Cover it with lots of lube, or if you don't have any lube you can use plenty of saliva.

The sphincter is the muscle on the outside of the anus. Press your finger against it for ten seconds so that it relaxes, and then carefully insert your finger. It can feel good to stretch the sphincter or to find the bulging prostate and press it. This kind of masturbation can take practice before you get it to work.

MIRROR

If you use a mirror when you jerk off, you can see what happens from an external perspective. One thing you can experiment with is the way things that are close to the mirror look bigger.

VACUUM CLEANER

Some comedies suggest that it feels like a blow job if you stick your dick into a vacuum cleaner. That's untrue, not least because a blow job is wet and the vacuum cleaner is dry. I advise against using a vacuum cleaner during masturbation, as many people have damaged their penis this way. The high pressure in the vacuum cleaner can damage the erectile tissue that swells with blood to give you an erection.

FANTASIZE

The brain is the body's most powerful sexual organ. It's where all your fantasies and desires are kept. Close your eyes and let yourself be carried away!

When it gets boring

Masturbating may not always be fun. One person who knows this feeling is Christian.

"I noticed I was jerking off just because, like an old habit. I did it every day when I didn't have anything else to do. Eventually I thought, *Why am I doing this?* And so I stopped," recalls Christian.

The break lasted two weeks. One day he felt properly horny and decided to jerk off.

"It was cool, it felt more enjoyable and I came a lot. Next day I jerked off again, thinking it would feel the same, but it didn't."

If, like Christian, you feel masturbating has become almost like a compulsion, something you *have* to do, it can be worth trying to break the cycle by taking a rest from jerking off, and thinking about what you did before, when it didn't feel like a compulsion.

If you feel that masturbating has become boring, you have to ask yourself whether you're really horny when you jerk off. If you're not horny, maybe you should leave it for a while?

If you always do the same thing and it's getting boring, you can try different ways of having solo sex. Perhaps something you've made up yourself? You probably have a lifelong relationship with masturbation ahead of you, as most people continue to jerk off even once they're in a relationship. So it would be a shame to get stuck in a rut instead of fully exploring and enjoying what solo sex has to offer.

PORN

In my early teens, I had no computer or smartphone, so I couldn't surf for porn. My first encounter with porn therefore came at night with a flickering cable channel. The picture came and went because we weren't paying the subscription.

I thought it was corny, a bit disgusting, and quite exciting to see the Italian men going at it with the heavily bleached-blonde women who moaned unnaturally loudly. The porn films were a long way from the sex I wanted to have, but I watched them anyway because they were the only game in town. Then I got my own computer and I was able to filter out what I didn't like, which was most of the porn out there.

Porn is not a new invention. Artists were painting images of people having sex several thousand years ago. Interest in such images has been around for a long time, but that doesn't mean everyone likes porn. Sometimes guys look at porn out of fascination or curiosity rather than horniness.

You can't enjoy all the porn out there. But if you find some porn that you like, it can make masturbation even more enjoyable. Porn is like a sexual encounter with no risk. You don't need to make an effort, you won't fall in love, and you don't need to think about using a condom.

Comes in many forms

There are many different kinds of porn because people have different tastes and fantasies. One type is the homemade porn filmed by amateurs. These people aren't trying to earn money by making porn. They may instead want to show themselves off or they might enjoy the sex more if they know it's being filmed. Sometimes amateur videos can be stolen and end up on the internet against the will of those involved. It is then illegal in many places to share this porn with other people.

Another type of porn is the animated kind. No real people are involved in this, which can be a relief—no one was harmed during the making of this porn. Since the porn is entirely made up, it can be far removed from reality. Some people have tentacles or angel wings or body parts the size of a house. There are communities where you can upload pornographic images you've drawn and comment on other people's pictures. If you're interested in Japanese animated porn, the words *hentai* (hetero porn), *yaoi* (gay porn) and *yuri* (lesbian porn) may be useful.

But not all porn is visual. There is also erotic fiction online that people write themselves and then post. Erotic fiction is the perfect way to find out what fantasies other people have, and you can write your own stories and publish them online.

There is a special type of erotic fiction called slash fiction. This involves characters from films or books having sex with each other. The name "slash" comes from the way the names of the characters who have sex with each other in the stories are written with a slash between them. For example, there's Aragorn/Legolas from *Lord of the Rings* or Harry/Ginny/Hermione from *Harry Potter*.

A world full of clichés

Movies often repeat the same stories. So you know, as soon as the romantic comedy begins, that the guy and the girl are going to get together. You know, when you see an action film, that the hero is probably going to be utterly beaten but will miraculously get up at the last moment and kill the villain. These stories are repeated because the filmmakers know they'll appeal to a broad audience. Porn films also repeat themselves.

A story often repeated in commercial hetero porn is one in which women are degraded. The girls are raped while the guys say horrible things to them and abuse them. In this case, the sex is not about a guy and a girl enjoying each other. Instead, it's about the guy taking what he wants, maybe as a punishment for the girl, because she's horny and is therefore labeled a slut.

> One in four guys don't like porn. Of those who do watch porn, a third are ashamed of doing so.*

Another recurring theme in commercial hetero and homo porn is the meeting of extreme bodies. Guys may have enormous dicks and girls sometimes may have breast implants. The girl's pussy may have been reduced through plastic surgery. Fake semen is even used so it looks like the guy is ejaculating more than he actually is. But there is no reason to think that sex would be better with a body like that.

Commercial porn also repeats the story of sex without a condom. Many porn stars have died of AIDS, but still many porn makers demand unsafe sex from their actors because it sells better.

Not a school for sex

I once talked to a guy who was tired of commercial porn.

"I don't get why it has to be like that. Can't the sex be a bit more like the sex people actually have?" he wondered.

The answer is no. The porn makers are not out to document how

---

*Source: Thomas Johansson and Nils Hammarén, *Koll på porr : skilda röster om sex, pornografi, medier och unga* [*Watching Porn: Different Voices on Sex, Pornography, Media and Youth*] (Stockholm: The State Media Council, 2006), 25–48.

people usually have sex or to educate everyone on how to have good sex. The main purpose of porn is to depict fantasies. So you should never think that sex has to be like in a porn film.

The fact that a film can be edited is a key reason why the sex in porn can be very different from sex in real life. Directors can cut out large sections so it looks as if the actors are having vaginal or anal intercourse without any warm-up first. If you do that in real life, it can be painful. It's also common to see a guy and a girl switching from anal sex to vaginal sex without changing the condom or washing their penis first. In reality, this could give the girl a urinary tract infection.

So basically, porn tells us nothing about how people actually have sex. But because commercial porn often repeats itself, it's easy to believe that real-life sex has to be like porn, otherwise the actors wouldn't have done it that way in film after film, would they? After one talk, a girl called Lisa came up to me and told me about her boyfriend.

"When we got together, I could tell that he'd watched too much porn. It was like he was repeating a load of things he'd seen guys do in porn films. I had to get across to him that sex wasn't about performing all kinds of tricks. Sex is for the two of us, not just him."

Watching porn doesn't automatically mean that you'll start behaving like the actors. But it's still good to keep in mind the realities of porn. The guy being sucked off may only have an erection because he's taken Viagra. The girl moaning away as she's being pounded might just be thinking about her next cigarette break. The people in the film are at work. And their job is to convince you that they're having a good time.

Exercise: Your fantasy

This exercise is for those who use porn.

Think about what your ultimate fantasy would be and write it down like a novel. Put in all the details from start to finish.

When you're done, compare your fantasy with the porn you watch: What's the same and what's different? Do you think the way the porn differs from your own fantasy is good or bad? If you think it's in any way bad, what can you do about it?

Being ashamed of porn

I once talked to my friend Mikael about porn. He said he was ashamed of the porn he looked at.

"I download films and watch them on my computer. It feels good while I'm doing it. But when I'm finished, I sometimes think, *What the hell have I been watching? What level have you sunk to?* I'm overcome by a bad feeling and I don't like myself," he explained.

"The main thing I don't like is the way the guys behave toward the girls. They're mean and completely brain dead, and they do things I think are really awful," he said.

It's not uncommon to feel ashamed of watching porn.

To ditch the shame, you have to differentiate between reality and fantasy. You might get aroused by a person being gangbanged in a porn film. If you were caught up in a group rape for real, you'd be disgusted. But what happens on-screen isn't real. The actors are only pretending to engage in rape. They are playing a trick on your mind, doing forbidden things to get your attention. So it's not that strange if you feel an urge to watch it.

Porn is fantasy, and in fantasy anything can happen and everything is allowed. The only thing you need to be able to defend is what you do in real life.

Why guys surf for porn*

68 percent to masturbate

63 percent to get horny alone

46 percent to relax

28 percent out of curiosity

23 percent to learn about sex

12 percent to get horny with a partner

Help, I'm addicted!

Many guys spend more time on porn than they think is healthy. It's just so easy to get hold of porn. With one click, you can escape the boring real world and enter the extreme porn world instead. There's so much

---

*Source: Sven-Axel Månsson, Ronny Tikkanen, Kristian Daneback, and Lotta Löfgren-Mårtenson, *Karlek och sexualitet pa internet* [*Youth and Sex on the Internet*] (Gothenburg and Malmo: Gothenburg University and Malmo University, 2003), 41.

porn out there that it can be hard to feel satisfied. Why should I come to this video, when there might be an even better video out there? So you can easily find yourself watching another video and then one more.

Porn loses some of its effect after you've seen it once. The first time, a video is hot. The next time the same guy watches the video, it's a little less interesting. After the third time, the video may start to feel boring. So the guy looks for more porn, where the porn actors are doing something new. A guy who began watching the film *Beautiful Sex with My Girlfriend* maybe half an hour later is watching scat sex in which seven dwarfs rape Snow White. And he can't understand how things got so out of hand!

Many guys get angry with themselves for this behavior. I notice guys increasingly believe they've become addicted to porn. I understand that people can become concerned, but being unhappy about watching porn is not the same as being addicted!

How not to feel bad about porn

- Write a porn diary, noting every time you look at porn. How were you feeling just before you started? For example, were you horny, bored, unhappy, or did you feel lonely? And after you watched the porn, did you feel mostly happy or unhappy?

- The porn diary will reveal the situations when you watch porn and feel unhappy afterward. Write a list of other things you can do in the same situation. If, for example, a guy often watches porn out of boredom, he has to write a

list of things to do when he's bored. He could call someone, do his homework at the library instead of at home, go
for a quick walk, join an orchestra for beginners, or clean
his room while dancing to good music.

- When you're in one of these typical situations where
you're thinking about watching porn and risk being
unhappy afterward, do one of the other things on your
list instead. Write down in your porn diary how it went.
The aim is not to stop looking at porn completely, as that
sets you up for failure. Instead, the aim is to reduce the
times you end up unhappy after watching porn.

THE MALE ROLE

No book for guys can ignore the actual role that guys are expected to
play in society. The male gender role is mainly what sets guys apart
from girls.

Imagine you meet a guy on the street. You've never seen him
naked, so you can't swear that he actually has a dick between his legs.
But still you're very sure that this person is a guy. That's because he is
sending out signals that say, "I'm a guy."

It might be his clothes, which may be loose fitting and show less
skin than girls' clothes. There are also particular colors and fabrics—
the colors may be dark and the fabric sturdy, not smooth as silk.
People can also signal that they are male by their hairstyle, not shav-
ing the hair on their legs and arms, and not wearing makeup.

But showing that you're a guy isn't just about appearance. The way you behave also counts. It may be about walking with big steps, sitting with your legs spread wide, or pitching your voice deep rather than high. Opinions can also be a way to show that you're a guy. You might think ice hockey is better than horseback riding, that being seen crying would be shaming, and that it's more important to win a competition than to look after someone who is unhappy.

All these things are different aspects of the male gender role. It's a system of unwritten rules that look slightly different, depending on where you live and how old you are. If you write down what you can and can't do if you want to look macho at your school, you'll get a rough picture of what the male gender role looks like where you are.

Part of the culture

The idea of what is masculine and what is feminine can feel so obvious that it's easy to believe it must be in our genes. But in fact it has nothing to do with genes or nature at all. Our view of what is masculine and feminine changes quickly over time, so it can't be genetic.

No one today finds it strange to see a woman walking around in trousers. A hundred years ago, people would have thought that was terrible and the sickest thing they'd seen in their life. Today it's perfectly normal for male performers to go up on stage and play the guitar. In the beginning, the guitar was a woman's instrument. But now no one is going to think *How strange that he's playing the guitar!*

What men show outwardly and what they actually feel inside may not always be the same. Two out of three men will not show signs of being sad or hurt.*

In two hundred years, guys will find pictures of you and me and think *What a stupid and weird style they had! They knew nothing about how to be a guy!*

These rapid changes come because the view of what is masculine and feminine is created by us humans. The male gender role is part of the culture, just like music. A few decades ago, radio stations played a lot of jazz, and today they play pop, rock, and hip-hop. Just as music tastes change, so does the idea about how guys and girls should behave.

Since the male gender role is part of the culture and not in our genes, it means we all have a choice. If you want to stick to the male gender role, you can. But if you don't want to, you can do things in an entirely different way.

Guys restrict each other

In practice, however, it isn't always easy to choose for yourself whether you want to play the male gender role.

I meet Mattias, who has had to switch schools a few times because he's been disruptive. He spends a lot of time with his gang of guys. Mattias says the guys in his gang like each other and would always

*Source: Hite, *The Hite Report on Male Sexuality*, 1091.

stand up for each other if there was trouble. But at the same time, they often say horrible things to each other as a joke.

"What would happen if one of the guys came to school one day in pink trousers?" I ask.

"That wouldn't be cool. We'd say he was a girl or call him gay. Not because he is gay, but because he has pink trousers on," says Mattias.

Even though they're good friends, they can't just do anything around each other.

"It's kind of too bad, actually. My friends and I have different views about some things, but you can't talk to them about it. There are things I can't say to them because they wouldn't understand," says Mattias.

It's common to act like Mattias and his friends: dissing other people when they don't stick closely enough to the male gender role. But when you're being hurtful to the person who dared swim against the tide, you're also being hurtful to yourself. In the long run, you're preventing yourself from being able to act and live the way you might want. Mattias tells me what he actually thinks about certain things, but he couldn't say anything to his friends because they'd mock him.

Half of all young men in high school have been called fag as an insult in the past year. The threat of getting a label that sticks keeps young men within the confines of the male gender role.*

---

*Source: Eva Witkowska, *Sexual Harassment in Schools: Prevalence, Structure and Perceptions* (Stockholm: Arbetslivsinstitutet [National Institute for Working Life], 2005), 26.

If you want to be able to choose for yourself whether to follow the male gender role, it's important to let other guys do what they want without commenting or being mean, no matter how unmacho or ridiculous you think they're being.

Following keeps us from growing

If you search for the words *Bonsai Kitten* online, you'll find an old internet hoax. Bonsai Kitten was a website with photographs of cats that had been squeezed into glass bottles. The website claimed to have started selling kittens like this. As the cats got bigger, they didn't have room to grow freely, and eventually they took on the same shape as the glass bottle.

Bonsai Kitten gives a good picture of what happens when you slavishly follow the male gender role, without listening to what you yourself really want. When you're a teenager, you're growing as a person. Personally, I changed friends, clothing styles, and opinions many times in just a few years before I finally found the person I was happy to be. It's stupid to stop yourself from trying different things as you grow. You can't grow beyond the restrictions of the male gender role if you think *I can't dress like that, I can't be friends with them, I can't do that*. The male gender role is like a Bonsai Kitten's glass bottle: It doesn't let you grow and take on your unique shape.

Another harmful aspect of the male gender role is that you're not supposed to show too much emotion. If you bottle up your emotions instead of dealing with them, in the long run you can end up feeling very bad, because your emotional life is squeezed out of shape like a Bonsai Kitten.

Listen to your inner voice. It's more important that you're happy with who you are. It matters less what other people think.

Power differences

As a group, guys have a special place in society, since boys and men have more power than girls and women. I don't mean that all guys have power, but if you compare all guys in one group with all girls in another, it's clear that guys have more power overall.

In school, that power can be about who dominates the classrooms, who forces their way to the head of the line, and who claims use of the football field, computers in the computer lab, or the pool table in the break room. Other things related to power are who gropes people and who scares other students.

The male gender role helps to create power differences because many guys consider it macho to act in a way that abuses others, such as hitting another guy or groping a girl. When guys play the stereotypical negative male gender role and do these things, it creates power differences. Some guys exert power over others.

I think guys should distance themselves from things in the male gender role that involve abusing other people: violence, threats, groping, taking up others' space, or making mean comments about gender, like calling someone a bitch or a slut. Do so for other people's sake, because they deserve to be treated with respect. But also for your own sake. Later on, I'll explain why you have a lot to gain from behaving respectfully.

The male gender role can make it more difficult for love to work out. Up to a quarter of couples who seek family therapy have problems rooted in gender roles.*

---

*Source: Estimate made by family therapist Anders Eklund Ramsten, DN, based on his experience.

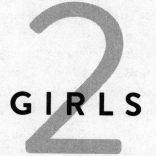

GIRLS

THE BODY

Now we're going on a guided tour of a girl's body.

If you're reading this book as a guy who mostly likes other guys, you might think you can skip this chapter. But I believe it's worth knowing what the other half of the population's bodies look like, whether or not you want to sleep with girls.

Imagine there is a naked girl lying next to you. You place your fingertips on her upper lip, where hair is growing, just like with guys. You slide your fingers down until you reach her throat. You can definitely feel a bump here, although it doesn't stick out as much as it does on many guys. This bump is commonly known as the Adam's apple.

Girls have the male sex hormone testosterone in their body, but not as much as guys do. In puberty, testosterone causes girls' voices to deepen. Their voices break, but usually not as noticeably as with guys. Move your hand down a little and you'll come to her breasts. Often one breast is slightly larger than the other, and they differ in shape. The size and shape of the breasts varies from person to person. Some girls have completely flat chests. It is often the case that the more subcutaneous (under the skin) fat a girl has on the body, the larger her breasts. However, there are many factors that can affect breast size, including genetics, medications, and intense athletic activity.

Just like with guys, hair grows on girls' chests. The amount and location varies.

Guys and girls can sometimes get stretch marks on their skin as they grow. The stretch marks may start out as blue-red lines, but they fade later. You can get stretch marks almost anywhere on the body, such as on the thighs and butt cheeks. It is not uncommon for girls to have stretch marks on their breasts.

Between the legs

Before we continue with the guided tour, I want to say that I use the word *pussy* to describe girls' entire genital area, including what is inside and outside the body. There are other words like snatch and muff, but *pussy* is the word I feel most comfortable with. I never use the word *pussy* as a swear word. For me it is the name of a body part; nothing more, nothing less.

Place your fingertips on her belly button. Follow the happy trail down until your fingers enter a bush of pubic hair. Just like with guys, the pubic hair is coarser than the hair on the head. The pubic hair runs out across the thighs and between the butt cheeks, like on guys.

Slide your fingers down through the hair to a mound of fatty tissue known as the pubic mound. When you get to the other side of the pubic mound, you're more or less in the place where the base of the penis sits on a guy. Here girls have a hood of skin, under which there is something that feels like a pearl.

This hood is just like a guy's foreskin, which protects and lubricates the glans. The pearl is the outer part of the clitoris: the clitoral shaft and the clitoral glans. If you pull back the hood, you can see the glans.

The bits that stick out are just a small part of the clitoris. Most of the clitoris is located inside the body.

If you follow the hood down on both sides, you'll find two flaps of skin that bulge out in various shapes. These are called the inner labia. In spite of their names, the inner labia are often partially visible over the outer labia. The outer labia are wrinkly and have hair, unlike the inner labia and clitoral hood.

If you part the inner labia, you'll see two openings. The top one is the urethra, the tube a girl pees through, and that may be hard to spot. It is so small that you can't feel it with your finger, and there is no way you'll accidentally stick anything up there. About an inch farther down is the vagina. Some people use the word *vagina* to describe girls' entire genital area, but in fact the vagina is just the "cave."

When a girl is not horny, the walls of the vagina touch each other and it would hurt her if you stuck a finger in. But the girl I want you to think about is turned on, so you can carefully push in a little bit of your finger. The vagina goes upward at an angle, and you can feel how the walls are uneven. Because this girl is horny, the vagina is wet inside. However, it's also moist when she's not horny.

How the pussy changes when she gets horny

- Girls get an erection. This means that blood flows down into the pussy. The clitoris grows, lifts, and gets hard. The labia grow and pull apart.
- The pussy becomes wet with a fluid that comes from the vagina and provides lubrication.
- The vagina becomes deeper and wider. The vagina swells and can feel as if it grows cushions around it.
- But these things don't *necessarily* mean that the girl is horny. Just like guys, girls sometimes get an erection without being horny.

The size of the vagina is not affected by how much sex a girl has. A vagina can't become "loose" from having many sexual partners. If the vagina feels tight, however, this is a sign that the girl is not aroused enough and then you need to take your finger out.

Just like with the dick, the pussy is darker than the rest of the body and the color can be patchy. The skin is also more wrinkled than in other places. If you compare different pussies, you'll notice that they vary in size and shape. The pussy can also have its own natural odor.

Exercise: Your own tour

Do the tour I've described, but with a hand on your own body.
This makes it easier to understand where the different parts
of the pussy are located.

If you're in a relationship with a girl or sleeping with her
and you really trust each other, you could ask if you can do
the tour on her instead.

Female ejaculation

When guys ejaculate, the sperm comes out at once in spurts. Girls
also produce a white fluid on orgasm, but it doesn't usually all come
out at the same time. It comes out of the urethra in waves and sometimes there is so little fluid that it goes unnoticed.

Sometimes, however, a lot might come in one go, as a stream. This
is called a squirting orgasm. It may not feel any different from her
other orgasms, it just looks different. It used to be thought that a girl
had peed herself when this happened, but now we know it's not pee
coming out of the urethra.

Girls' ejaculate comes from female prostate glands that are not unlike a guy's prostate. The difference is that guys have one large prostate whereas girls have several small glands arranged around the
urethra.

Girls and guys are a lot alike

When I started learning about the pussy, I found it hard going. There were so many body parts that were new to me, they had all these new names, and I didn't really know what they were for.

> The clitoris is longer than the penis in its soft state. But most of the clitoris is located inside the body.

But in fact there is no mystery about the pussy. All fetuses start out the same in their mother's belly, whether they are going to end up being a boy or a girl. The pussy and the dick thus develop from the same basic origin, which is why they both have similar parts. Below you can see what your genitals equate to in a female, which will hopefully make it easier to understand a girl's body.

Penis	Clitoris
Glans on penis	Glans on clitoris
Foreskin	Clitoral hood and inner labia
Skin of the scrotum	Outer labia
Testicles	Ovaries inside the body
Male prostate	Female prostate glands

IDEALS

Girls are always being told that they aren't good enough as they are and have to change. Sometimes it is communicated openly, like in women's magazines that cover dieting and makeovers. But the message can also be more hidden.

For example, the lower half of a bikini is often triangular. And yet you'll never see girls' pubic hair in the bikini ads. As if girls' pubic hair grows in perfect little triangles! A girl who puts on a bikini may notice her pubic hair poking out, which didn't happen for the model in the ad. And so she gets the signal that her hair growth is somehow wrong. She needs to change to fit into the image of what the advertising industry tells us a girl in a bikini should look like.

Often the ideal is presented as normal and something that girls achieve effortlessly. When a movie shows a girl who has just woken up, she's usually lying in bed with perfect makeup and hair. As if girls were born ready-styled.

"You have to meet the criteria for what a girl looks like before you're counted as a proper girl," as my friend Johanna puts it.

A girl who doesn't make the expected changes, who doesn't wax or wear makeup, therefore risks being seen as unfeminine.

There's nothing wrong with waxing or wearing makeup if that's what you want, no matter what your gender. Lots of people enjoy it. The problem is with the perpetuation of the ideal, which makes many girls feel as if they don't have any choice. Feeling like they can't live up to all these demands can affect the health of some girls.

No girl can ever completely live up to the ideal because it's inhuman to never sweat, get acne, or age. If you diss girls when they don't follow the ideal, there is therefore a risk that no girl will dare show you who she really is. The ideal then becomes a wall that prevents you from getting to know girls better.

Oppression of the pussy

Maybe the strangest idea of what girls should be like is that they mustn't have . . . a pussy.

Think about it! Are there any statues of naked women where you live? If so, do they have pussies? Statues of naked women are almost always flat in the genital area—they don't have any sex. Statues of men, on the other hand, are allowed to have a penis.

Go to the personal hygiene aisle in a supermarket and you will find perfumed panty liners. The message is clear: Pussies mustn't smell of pussy; they must smell of perfume! If, on the other hand, you go to a sports store to buy a jockstrap, will that be perfumed with wildflowers and cinnamon? No, of course not.

> "Sundays are an unfeminine day. You don't shower, your hair hangs limply, you don't shave between your legs. It's quite hard work being feminine all the time; you don't always have the energy. You just can't be bothered. Sometimes you just want to take things easy."*

*Source: Fanny Ambjörnsson, *I en klass för sig : genus, klass och sexualitet bland gymnasietjejer* [*In a Class of Their Own: Gender, Class and Sexuality among High School Girls*] (Stockholm: Ordfront Forlag, 2010).

All this antipussy feeling has gone so far that it has even spread to porn. Many female porn stars have plastic surgery on their pussy to make it smaller. They cut away large chunks of their sensitive labia and then have to pretend that they're having a good time in the films.

The oppression of the pussy is bad news. It means guys know less about pussies and girls are less able to feel happy with their bodies. In the long term, both these aspects can make it more difficult for girls to enjoy sex.

We need the pussy to be more visible on our streets and squares until everyone realizes that the pussy is fine as it is.

SEXUALITY

I'm sitting with Carro, Lana, and Sara at a café, talking about horniness. As we drink tea, I recall how I saw girls when I was younger. I had been fed the image of girls not being as sexual as guys. When I visit schools today, I notice that the guys have often been fed the same image. So we might as well sort this out once and for all.

"Are girls as horny as guys?" I ask.

"Yes, definitely," say the girls around the table.

"But it also depends on the person. Some girls are maybe not as horny. But some guys aren't all that horny either," says Lana.

Sara thinks the big difference is that girls' horniness doesn't get as much attention as guys'.

"We don't go on about it the way guys do. Guys have loud conversations about porn and masturbation in the classroom. It's almost as if guys have to show the whole school how horny they are. Girls aren't supposed to be open like that," says Sara.

"Exactly! A guy can say 'Suck my dick' to someone, but how often are you going to get an angry girl saying 'Lick my pussy' to a guy?" says Carro.

The girls laugh.

"Do girls have to be in love to get horny?" I ask.

"What? No! Anyone can make you horny. It could be a singer or just someone hot who you pass on the street," says Lana.

Girls masturbate

When we get onto the subject of masturbation, Sara recalls something that happened to her at a different school when she was about thirteen or fourteen. It was in a biology lesson, where the class had been split into two groups, with the girls all in one room and the boys in another. The idea was for the students to talk about masturbation.

"A classmate told us about a girl in the neighboring school who masturbated every day. The classmate said she thought it was disgusting that the girl masturbated, and all the others agreed, saying 'God, that's so disgusting!'"

"What did you do?" I asked.

"I went along with everyone else and made faces to show that it was the most horrible thing I'd ever heard. But that wasn't true. I masturbated and I actually didn't see anything wrong with it. But we had to pretend, even though there weren't any teachers or boys around listening to us," says Sara.

I ask whether she believed the classmates who claimed they didn't masturbate.

"No, of course I didn't. I thought most of them masturbated just like I did. But I wasn't entirely sure. Maybe there was something wrong with me?"

Carro, Lana, and Sara feel that society sometimes seems to have a problem with girls owning their own sexuality.

"Girls are expected to be like in the fairy tales. A princess sitting in a tower with her hands firmly on top of the covers, waiting for a boy to travel around the world to come and get her. Girls are not expected to take matters into their own hands, even though they are perfectly capable. Our sexuality is not welcome," says Carro.

How they pleasure themselves

Just like guys, girls masturbate in many different ways. It's common for girls to stroke their whole pussy or rub against something, like a pillow. They may also rub the clitoral hood backward and forward over the clitoral glans, like the way guys who are uncircumcised jerk off. Girls mainly get an orgasm by stroking the clitoral glans and putting external pressure on the parts of the clitoris that are inside the body.

Girls may also masturbate by inserting a finger or something else into the vagina. And it's not only the genitals that have sensitive spots. Like guys, girls can masturbate by touching their butt, stomach, thighs, and the rest of the body.

The clitoral glans is more sensitive than the head of the penis. It has twice as many nerve endings as the glans penis.

When I ask the girls in the café whether it's hard to bring yourself to orgasm when masturbating, they say it depends whether you know what you're doing.

"You can do it in as little as a minute. But sometimes you might want to draw it out and not orgasm as quickly. Or you can keep going for a long time and have multiple orgasms," says Lana.

"Some can find it more difficult to climax than others. But it gets easier when you're a few years older and have been doing it for a while," says Sara.

On average, girls start having sex earlier than guys. But girls risk getting a worse reputation if they talk openly about their sexuality and sex. Guys have less to lose when talking about sex. Perhaps this explains why guys' sexuality takes up more space in society.*

NO BLOOD DURING SEX

Research into girls' bodies is a bit behind the curve. For a long time, people have fallen back on myths rather than facts. Perhaps the most famous myth about girls' bodies is the myth of the hymen. If you've heard of the hymen before, you've probably heard about a membrane

*Source: Margareta Forsberg, *Ungdomar och sexualitet* [*Youth and Sexuality*] (Stockholm: Statens Folkhälsoinstitut, 2006), 14–21.

or string inside the girl that breaks and bleeds when she has vaginal intercourse for the first time. But this isn't what it is at all.

Imagine you stand with your face between the girl's legs, pulling her labia apart and looking into her vagina. The first thing you'll see is a membrane of soft tissue with the opening into the vagina in the middle, and this soft tissue is the hymen. The shape of the opening in the hymen is different on different girls. Because the hymen is able to stretch, just like the rest of the vagina, most girls can have sex for the first time without bleeding or feeling pain, while others might experience both. But the most common result of consenting sex filled with positive emotions will be no blood and no pain. Some girls, however, have a hymen shaped in a way that can get a rupture if she has intercourse. It can hurt, causing a slight burning feeling, but it usually doesn't bleed much because the membrane has very few blood vessels.

But you can't tell if someone has had sex or not based on the hymen because each one is unique in its shape! As a guy, if you've checked in the showers, you know that not all dicks look alike. It's the same with vaginas, everyone's is different.

Men and women have believed that the hymen worked as a virginity detector for a long time, and this has created problems. Across the ages and around the world, women have had to fake bleeding on their wedding night in various ways. And because no one has unmasked this hymen myth, it has lived on.

"But I've heard that doctors can fix the hymen if the girl is at risk of being murdered!" said one guy once, when I explained about this.

Sometimes if a girl is in mortal danger, a stitch may be sewn into the hymen tissue so that when the girl has sex, the stitch will come out and cause her to bleed. Even a procedure like this, however, can't guarantee bleeding.

There is, of course, a real reason why this myth about the hymen exists. It has made girls afraid to have sex before marriage. The myth has basically made it easier for parents and men to control girls' sexuality. But you simply can't compare two girls' vaginas and identify who has had sex and who hasn't. It's impossible, because vaginas vary so much.

It doesn't have to be painful

Another side to the myth of the hymen is the claim that girls always find vaginal sex painful the first time because the hymen is torn. But there are no nerve endings in the hymen, so sex doesn't have to be painful, not even the first time.

"When I found having sex with a guy painful, I thought that was just how it was supposed to be. But afterward I realized that I'd had fingers in my vagina many times without experiencing any pain. Why should it be painful just because I was sleeping with a guy?" asks Elin, who has sex with both guys and girls.

"I put a finger inside her and felt a fleshy cord bisecting her vagina like a tennis net. This was her hymen."*

---

*Source: Neil Strauss, *The Game* (New York: ReganBooks, 2005), 210, in which pickup artist Strauss recalls the girls he has slept with. But it turns out he doesn't know much about women's bodies and probably made up at least one of his many sex stories.

The myth of the hymen may also have stuck around so that girls will put up with bad sex that hurts. It makes them believe that sex has to be like that, so it's completely OK to suffer painful sex, when in fact they could be having pain-free sex every time.

You can't tell if she has had sex

OK, so the hymen isn't a virginity detector. How do we explain the fact that some girls do actually find sex painful the first time?

In almost every case, it's because you're doing it wrong. You might push too hard, be nervous, not feel ready (lubricated), or go at it too quickly. The first time doesn't have to be like that. Later in the book we'll look at what you can do if you want to have sex with a girl in a way that both of you enjoy.

MENSTRUATION

Now I'm going to admit something embarrassing. It's about the first time I slept with a girl who was menstruating. When we were about to get into bed, she said: "There's just one thing. I'm on my period right now. I hope it's not a problem if I end up bleeding a bit on your sheet?"

I froze. In my head I could see myself waking up the next morning with the sheets drenched in blood. The blood was making my pajama bottoms stick to my legs. The red liquid was cold and its strong smell of iron was overwhelming my senses.

"What's wrong?" the girl asked.

She could tell from the look on my face that I was terrified. Terrified of the menstrual monster. When I told her how I felt, she said I was prejudiced. And it was true, I was prejudiced! I had lived my whole life among women at home and at school. But none of them had talked about their period. The only ideas about menstruation I had to fall back on were the ones I'd cooked up in my own head; in other words, my prejudices.

We went to sleep.

When we got up in the morning, there was a tiny dark-red spot of menstrual blood on my sheet.

"Was that it?" I asked her.

The menstrual monster attacks!

Imagine what it would be like if men menstruated instead of women. Periods would no doubt be another subject to brag about in the locker room.

"I'm bleeding so heavily. It's just gushing out!"

But because we live in a society where the pussy has to be kept behind closed doors, menstruation has instead become shameful. When tampons and panty liners are advertised on TV, they don't actually show any menstrual blood (menses), even though that's exactly what these products are designed to absorb. Instead they replace the blood with a fresh blue liquid.

> Menses is mucus and blood that the body flushes out if the female has not been impregnated during ovulation. The menses varies in color and can fall anywhere in the range between red, brown, and black. It can be runny or thick.

All the propaganda about the menstrual monster leaves guys with a belief that the whole of the girl changes when she's on her period, kind of like how a full moon transforms some people into werewolves. If a girl has period pains, then she may not feel on top of the world exactly. But if a girl gets angry, it's not because she's menstruating. It's because something has happened to make her angry. Like someone being a dick.

Many guys have asked me whether you can have sex with a girl who is on her period. And the answer is yes, of course you can. If you both want to have sex and you're not going to freak out if you get a little menstrual blood on your fingers or dick, you can carry on as normal. Lay a towel underneath you to avoid getting blood on the sheet. The menstrual monster is not going to eat you alive.

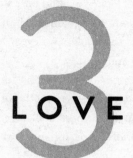

LOVE

IN LOVE

The teacher began the lesson by drawing a full glass of water on the board. He said there was a little more water in the glass than there was actually space for. "So why didn't the water overflow?" he asked the classroom in the faint hope that someone would put their hand up.

I looked around the cold science room. I was looking for a Special Person (SP) who wasn't there. SP was never late for school, so this probably meant that SP was sick. I wouldn't be seeing SP for several days, or maybe even a whole week!

I rested my head heavily in my hands. As the lesson ground on, I thought about how my body felt. My brain was mushy, my body weak. Maybe I was sick too? Maybe it was best if I also stayed home for the week?

And then the door opened. SP burst in and, short of breath, apologized to the teacher. SP looked around for an empty seat at the back of the class and sat down. I brightened up and little electric shocks swept over my skin. In the blink of an eye, I had gone from a sickly feeling to being happy and healthy.

Love is powerful. It can make you feel sick or alive. It can make you behave strangely, see new things as a matter of life and death, or give you a stomachache. But maybe best of all, love can make you feel that you're not the most important person in the world, that you're not the center of the universe.

There are many different kinds of love. You can love a friend, love a pet, or love someone in your family. For many people a friend, parent, or sibling can be just as important as or more important than a girlfriend or boyfriend. Many single people think they have the perfect life and don't need a partner. There's no reason for romantic love to be any more important than the other love in your life.

Affection at a distance

Sometimes you fall in love with someone who is far removed from you or you may never even have spoken to—like a hot person you sometimes see in town, or a singer or actor. Being in love from a distance is a positive thing because it makes your body feel good and allows you to dream. At the same time, you avoid the risk of getting hurt.

> "Frisson. Of danger? Of passion? Either/or. Take
> your pick: danger in b., passion in me. Both, probably.
> Which knowledge gave me a frisson of frisson. With
> which tingle in the testes I drifted into dozy cozy
> daydream slumber."*

There seems to be an attitude in society that at some point in your teenage years it stops being OK to be in love from a distance, and you can only be in love with people closer to you. This is because many see love from a distance as training for "real" love and don't attach any value to the former. But I think you should continue being in love with people from a distance for as long as you want. It's actually a cool thing that doesn't do anyone any harm.

Being in love from a distance also doesn't mean you can't fall in love with people closer to you and get together with them.

Longing for love

I remember times when I longed for love. I wasn't longing for any one person in particular, I just wanted to be in love and going out with someone. This longing is hardly surprising. There can be many benefits to being in a relationship. You have someone to cuddle when you want intimacy. Someone to sleep with who means more to you than a casual friend with benefits. And you can talk about things you

---

*Source: Aidan Chambers, *Breaktime and Dance on My Grave* (London: Definitions, 2007), 96.

wouldn't dare discuss with your friends for fear of being mocked mercilessly.

If you do long for love, you may sometimes wonder, *Why don't I have anyone? What's wrong with me?* But there is no point in thinking like that, because there's no real explanation as to why certain people are together and others aren't. Many of my male friends who are good-looking, kind, and funny are single despite being real catches. Being a good guy isn't enough. It's all down to chance whether you meet the person you click with. Sometimes you have to be happy with your single life before you find someone.

Love in real life

As with so many things, there is a difference between the image of love and love in the real world. In the movies, love is about two people finding each other and finding contentment. Then the movie ends when they are still newly in love and super happy.

But in reality, you're not going to be that happy and drunk in love all the time. You were a fully rounded person when you entered into the relationship and you will continue to be so. The world will continue to turn. All the baggage you took into the relationship remains. If you had problems with your family, with school, or with yourself, they will still be there. Nobody but you, not even your partner, can solve your problems.

Being together doesn't necessarily mean always being happy. Nor is loving someone always easy. You'll fight and cry and battle hard to make the relationship work. This doesn't mean there is anything wrong with your love. On the contrary, it may be because you love each other that you fight.

Nothing has made me grow in my own life as much as love. It is healthy to have someone other than yourself to think about.

FLIRTING

As usual I was late for school. It was Valentine's Day, which I'd completely forgotten. Everything was normal in the classroom except that my friend Sandra was holding a bouquet of red roses. I sat next to her and asked who she'd gotten them from. She said Joel.

"Joel? You mean Joel in our class?" I said. She nodded.

"It was just before the lesson. He came up to me by the lockers and held out this bouquet. At first I didn't get that they were for me. He was absolutely red in the face. He said he was in love with me and then he walked off," said Sandra.

I looked around the classroom and it was true, Joel wasn't there.

"So. What are you going to do?" I asked.

"When we've finished, I'll have to call and thank him for the flowers but say that I don't feel the same way. I thought we were just friends."

"But did you know he was in love with you?"

"No, it was a complete surprise. I had no idea," said Sandra.

It was also a surprise to me. You'll often notice when someone is interested in you, but Joel hadn't shown any signs.

It was brave of Joel to go up and say what he did to Sandra. But maybe not the most tactical approach. If you surprise someone by telling them you're in love, there's a risk that you'll frighten them off if they can't handle such strong emotions all at once. Imagine how you would react if someone came out of nowhere and said they were in love with you!

Instead of saying how you feel, you can show your interest through the way you act.

Dare to make contact

We all live in our own bubbles. When you're in school or at a party, you divide people up into two categories: those you know and those you don't know. You look at and listen to your friends. Everyone else ends up more in the background, and you hardly notice them.

The same is true of the way other people see you. As long as you're one of the people "I don't know," you'll stay in the background. And that makes it difficult for anyone to see you and be interested in you. It's much easier if you make contact and start talking to each other. In that way the other person can get to know you and decide if they like you.

If you get nervous easily, try not to make a big thing of going up and talking. You're just talking, you're not going down on one knee and proposing! When you talk, you may even find that you don't like the person after all. See it as a way to check the person out rather than trying to get together. Sometimes it may feel easier if you come up with a reason to make contact. You could ask a person to take a picture of you and your friend on your phone, for example.

Another way to make contact is to get in with the whole group that the person is part of. When you feel secure within the group, you can then focus on talking to the person you're interested in.

Get the conversation going

If you feel shy or nervous about going up and talking to someone, it can be good to have one or two icebreakers up your sleeve. An icebreaker is a topic of conversation you can talk about for a bit, preferably one that comes in the form of a question.

If you know something about the person you want to talk to or you have something in common, that should offer you some quite natural icebreakers. If you go to the same school, you can say, "Don't you think our history teacher is in a good mood lately? Do you think she's in love?" If you know the person is interested in fashion, you could say, "I'm thinking of buying my big brother a sweater for his birthday. Do you think the choice of brand is always important?"

So an icebreaker is all about opinions. A factual question like "What's the capital of Bulgaria?" works better in Mastermind than when you're flirting.

Once you've exhausted the icebreaker, you'll hopefully no longer feel shy and you can talk about other things without it feeling strange that the two of you are talking to each other.

Show interest

Of course it doesn't have to be you who makes the first move. Sometimes the other person is the one who takes the plunge and starts up a conversation. If you're also interested, it can be a good idea to show it. Smile, try to maintain eye contact, and ask follow-up questions related to what the person is talking about so they feel you're finding it interesting. If you're really pleased the person has struck up a conversation with you, you can say so. You have nothing to lose if the other person is the one who took the first step. And if you're going somewhere, you can invite the person to join you.

Remember that you're not obliged to give anything back just because a person pays you some attention or buys you a beer, for example.

The effect of alcohol

Many people are drunk the first time they make out or have sex with someone. This is because many feel braver when they've been drinking. It can feel easier to make contact and talk, which is of course a good thing.

But for your love life and sex life to work in the long term, you also have to have the courage to do things without alcohol. Many guys can't summon up the courage to dance or talk unless they're drunk, and that's a problem, because it means you have to be drunk every time you want that courage. If you usually resort to alcohol, try dancing and talking to people when you're sober. If it feels hard, you could possibly even pretend to be drunk. In the long term, you'll benefit from plucking up the courage, because you can get to know people better and have more enjoyable sex when you're sober. In addition, people make smarter decisions when they're sober.

When you make contact with another person, it can feel easier if you're drunk, because then you may forget that you lack confidence. But if you want to get together with someone, you also have to meet and like each other when you're both sober. If the person you're interested in only kisses you or sleeps with you when they're drunk, that's a bad sign. You should also remember that if someone is blind drunk, they can't consent to having sex. The law in the U.S. says that no matter what they say, if they are drunk, they aren't giving consent. So if you meet someone who's just too drunk, don't sleep with them, because you would be taking advantage of a person in need. Instead, be a friend. Take them home (their home!), make sure they're OK, and leave them your number. That way, you can meet again under better conditions.

Alcohol can sometimes make it easier to connect with people, but not always. Many people become dull, annoying, and stupid when they drink. That pushes away people who would otherwise have liked them in a sober state.

If you do drink, try not to get blind drunk, because that can easily give a bad impression, particularly if the other person is sober or less drunk than you. Bear in mind that nothing can ruin a pickup as effectively as you throwing up.

Getting to know each other

Try to spend as much time as possible with the person you're interested in. In this way you get to see whether there is any chemistry between you. If the person lives in your neighborhood, you can seize every natural opportunity you get. If they and a few others are off to hang out somewhere, tag along. If they and a few friends are going to the movies, say you really want to see that film too.

It's also good for just the two of you to meet up. At first, plan to get together for an everyday activity so that you're joining in with something the person would be doing anyway. They're just doing it with you today. If the person is off to the H&M sale, go with them. If they're waiting for a bus, help them kill time until the bus comes.

That way it doesn't feel like a date, which reduces any nervousness.

But make sure you're clear with them about what you want! If the other person thinks you just want to be friends, they might only be able to see you that way. And once that picture of you has taken hold, it's difficult to shift. Sometimes guys talk about getting into the "friend zone" and get frustrated because they think that girls will never want to go out with "nice" guys. But being nice isn't the problem; the problem is not being clear about your intentions.

You have to indicate that you're interested, even though this increases the risk of being rejected. The easiest way to show you're interested is by saying something nice about the person or making casual physical contact.

Casual physical contact is when you touch the other person in a nice way even though it's not necessary. If you touch the person on the arm to get their attention or remove a leaf from the person's jacket, you're making casual physical contact. If the person makes casual physical contact back, you know you're on the right track. But if the person seems to feel you're invading their space, you must immediately back off and stop!

To avoid any misunderstanding, I want to stress that casual physical contact is not sexual. Touching someone's shoulder shows that you like them. Touching someone's ass shows that you want a kick in the balls.

Meet on social media

By far the easiest way of making contact with new people is through social media and apps. You instantly get access to thousands of people without even having to get up off the sofa. When you're chatting with a person instead of talking to them face-to-face, there is a little distance between you. Many people like this distance because it makes them less nervous. You also get a little extra thinking time, which is good if you find it hard to know how to flirt.

How to interpret signals

- Smiling, nice comments, and casual physical contact mean that she, he, or they like you.
- If the person asks what you think or asks about you and your life, that person is interested in finding out more about you.
- If the person is always around wherever you are, they enjoy your company.
- If the person you're interested in never seems to have time to meet up, doesn't call or text, and doesn't pay you any attention, this means the interest is not mutual or they're just playing you.
- Don't overinterpret every detail. People don't think about every tiny thing they say or do. The bigger picture shows whether or not the person is into you, not the small stuff.

Unfortunately, this distance also has its downside. Many people forget that the person they're chatting with is real and has feelings. This makes some people really unkind when they interact online. They write mean things and then don't feel bad about it because they can't see how upset the other person is. A good rule of thumb is to treat people with the same respect at a distance as you would face-to-face.

If you started exchanging messages with someone you find interesting, it's good to take some kind of step to reduce the distance between you. You could try a phone call or video chat, for example. That way you both know the person you've been messaging is real. Now actually meeting up is not such a leap.

If you want to meet, it's a good idea to suggest a place where there are other people around. Ask if they want to grab a bite to eat and then go for a walk in the sunshine. Having people around puts you on safer ground in case the person turns out to be nuts. It also makes the other person feel more secure. If instead you meet in some deserted place that's straight out of a slasher movie, don't be surprised if your date is a bit nervous.

Is he into guys?

If you're interested in a girl, there's quite a good chance that she likes guys. But if it's a guy you're interested in, there's only a one in ten chance that he likes guys. Before you put too much effort in, you therefore may want to establish whether or not he likes guys.

You should, obviously, look out for classic clues: he has a rainbow decal on his backpack, he really doesn't care what hetero guys think about him, or his ex-boyfriend wants to kill you. But if there are no obvious signs, you can try saying something relevant to the gay world.

If there's a youth club for the LGBTQ community where you live, you can ask what he thinks about the place. You can also ask about films and series with gay characters. What does he think about the film *Moonlight* or the anime series *Yuri!!! on Ice*? You could also bring up gay dating apps.

If the guy looks confused and doesn't know what you're talking about, it's probably the case that he's not into other guys. If he was, he would have sought out venues, films, and websites on that theme! You can just change the conversation and pretend nothing happened.

Not all hope is lost, however. He may never have realized that he likes guys until he met you.

If you want other guys to have a chance to flirt with you, it helps if you're open about liking guys or give some kind of signal, like a rainbow decal.

Cards on the table

Sometimes you can end up in a game of cat and mouse, with things always being hinted at. There are lingering looks and coy smiles. You spend time together, but nothing ever happens. At this point it's worth confronting the person, telling them how you feel, and asking them how they feel.

Otherwise, there is a risk that you'll just get stuck in the game. After all, getting noticed and validated is cool. The person you like might just enjoy being the center of attention and have no intention of getting together with you. Or maybe they've been waiting months for you to take the first step, as they can't pluck up the courage to do it themselves. In this case it is worth putting all your cards on the table. It may or may not go the way you want it to. In the worst case, you can at least move on and focus on other people.

Getting turned down

Here comes a harsh truth. Not everyone is going to like you. Not everyone is going to fall in love with you. Not everyone wants to sleep with you. Of the people you meet each day, you probably consider very few of them to be prime hookup material, don't you? The same is true for them. Most people who meet you won't want to go out with you. No matter how hot, smart, and funny you are.

It is therefore unavoidable that you are going to suffer rejection at some point. Being turned down has nothing to do with who you are, and it doesn't necessarily mean you've done anything wrong.

Being rejected hurts, but it's nothing to be afraid of. The more times it happens, the less serious it feels. It gets easier to dust yourself off and not let it affect your self-esteem. You can't click with everyone. But take a no seriously. If someone doesn't want to be with you, let it go immediately.

If you've been rejected many times, I'd like to congratulate you. Getting a no means you're putting yourself out there. If you've been rejected, it means you dared to try and dared to take risks. That's a good thing! It's better to be rejected a hundred times than never to be rejected at all, because that means you haven't even tried.

KISSES

I had a friend in school who was going out with a girl he wanted to kiss, but he had never kissed anyone before. We hung out at his house and talked about what he should do. Unfortunately I was no help because I'd never kissed anyone either. What's more, I was even more shy than my friend. In the end he set a deadline by which he would kiss her, but that date came and went and he still hadn't managed it.

My first time kissing was easier because it came as a surprise. One day at a youth club in town I saw a person I hadn't seen before. They looked at me too, and there was an exciting tension between us as we both looked at each other with interest. Because I was a coward, it fell to the other person to come up to me and say hi.

We sat on a sofa and chatted. I think it was quite difficult to take in what we said because the tension between us was electric. It's the chemistry that happens when you're interested and you know the other person is too!

The person took out some hand cream and rubbed it into their hands. I said, "Taking hand cream out with you is smart. I should do that. Look, my hands are so dry."

"Here, give me your hands," they said, and they smoothed cream over my hands. Then we kissed. It was wet and the feeling of another person's tongue against mine was very different than what I'd imagined.

Step-by-step: How to work up to a kiss

1. Say something nice about the other person, so they understand that you like them.
2. Make casual physical contact with the other person's body. For example, you could say that the person has a cool top on and hold them by the arm for a little while.

This builds up a physical closeness between you, so it doesn't feel like the kiss comes out of nowhere. This is exactly what the person did to me, when they rubbed hand cream into my hands.

3. Lean toward the person, but don't go all the way. Read the other person's reaction! If they back away, you should back away too. If they lean forward or part their lips and close their eyes, go for it!

Kissing

There are two parts to a kiss. One part is the tongue-to-tongue contact. You can lick the other person's tongue a little or let your tongues wriggle around in circles. All you have to do is take it easy and go with what feels right and it'll go great.

The other part is what you do with your lips. You can kiss each other lightly in between the deeper kisses or stroke the other person's lips with your own.

The joy of kissing is that there are so many different ways of doing it. You don't have to do the same thing every time. The best thing is to not think about what you're doing and let the kissing take care of itself. Try closing your eyes and losing yourself in the kissing, to the point where there's nothing else in the world but the two of you.

What to think about when kissing

- A kiss doesn't have to last for minutes on end. Sometimes the pleasure can come from kissing and stopping and kissing again, so you pause for breath.
- You don't need to force your tongue particularly far into the other person's mouth. At worst, it can feel unpleasant and suffocating for the other person. Try to meet halfway with your tongues.
- It's best to breathe through your nose rather than your mouth.
- Try not to drench the other person's lips with saliva, as they might not like it.
- If you have stubble on your face, the other person might find it prickly. Try to keep your face fairly still.
- When you're kissing each other, you can touch the other person's neck and stroke their chin or scalp.

NICE GUYS

When I was in secondary school, there was a certain type of guy that got all the attention from the girls. It was the kind of guy who always played the bad boy. They spat indoors, sometimes boasted about having committed a crime, and enjoyed bullying younger students.

There's even a harmful stereotype that has circulated online, calling that kind of guy a "Chad" and any girl who likes him a "Stacy." These memes have surfaced on forums run by guys calling themselves *Incels* (short for "involuntary celibates," who blame women for not wanting to sleep with them) and have been used to promote violence against women. This might seem extreme, but it's an example of the same idea taken too far.

It seems that little has changed since my day in many respects, and you don't have to go to the dark corners of the internet to see how. Often when I'm out in schools now, boys complain that girls don't want nice guys. But is that really true? When I've conducted interviews, I've talked to girls about this. And everyone I've spoken to agrees: Girls want nice guys.

Nasim is one of the girls I spoke to. She says there's a certain type of girl who attracts attention from all the guys.

"They dress a bit sexier and maybe wear more makeup than other girls to get noticed. These girls go out with guys who also do things to get noticed, guys who act out and go around groping girls. But the vast majority of the girls at school aren't like that. The problem is that no guy ever comes up and talks to the other girls," says Nasim.

According to Nasim, the blame in fact lies with guys who only want to go out with a particular kind of girl. But in one way, Nasim agrees with the guys I've spoken to.

"Guys who take up space and can't keep their hands to themselves become the center of attention. You know they're there because you can see them. You've got no idea who the other guys are because you've never had anything to do with them. I think if nice guys talked to girls more, girls would discover them and maybe want to spend more time with them."

Start getting noticed

Just because you're a nice guy who likes girls, it doesn't mean you have to stay in the background. There are smarter ways of getting noticed than groping girls and smashing windows.

- Talk to all the girls, just as friends. This makes it easier later on to talk to girls you're interested in.
- Try to say hi and be nice to everyone in your environment, whether the person is super popular, a complete nerd, or somewhere in between. Talk to people in other groups. Because you've made contact, others will find it easier to come up to you and talk.
- Get yourself some female friends. If you become good friends, they will lower their guard and then you'll see that girls can be just like guys. The mysterious veil will be lifted, and you'll find it easier to understand women.
- Notice people who don't get noticed. In my experience, the quiet ones are often the ones with interesting things to say.
- Don't judge guys who act tough to be the center of attention or girls who like this type of guy. They no doubt have their reasons for behaving like this. And you can't know the whole story. Maybe the tough guy is kind and gentle when he's alone with his girlfriend.

GOING OUT

When you're going out with someone, there are two things that are worth talking about as soon as it feels comfortable to do so. First you need to define your relationship. Are you together? Are you dating?

Or are you just fooling around? So many times I've seen friends enter into a relationship without defining what they're doing, and a few weeks later one of the people involved ends up hurt because they thought it was more serious than it actually was.

The second thing you need to talk about is what rules apply in your relationship. What do you agree that you can do with other people while you're together? People tend to have different views on this point. Some think it's OK to make out with someone. Some think it's fine to also sleep with other people. Others think you shouldn't do anything at all with others. If you don't talk about this, someone might get hurt.

Does having to talk and set ground rules sound like hard work? Get used to it. Going out with someone relies heavily on talking and understanding each other.

Talk to each other

A typical problem in relationships comes after an initial period of being together day and night, when one of you begins to feel suffocated. You want to hang out with your friends and spend time on your interests. You want to stay together, but you don't think the relationship should entirely take over your life.

The wrong way to deal with the problem is to continue being together 24-7 against your will or to pretend that you're ill and have to stay at home, so you can sneak out and meet your friends. The right way to tackle the issue is to sit down and talk. Both of you can talk about what you feel and think, so you can negotiate your way to a solution that feels acceptable to you both.

Masses of problems large and small crop up in relationships, particularly if you're together for a long time. It can relate to anything from how often you talk on the phone to who decides what you do together. If you can keep the channels of communication open, you can solve the problems as they arise. But if you don't talk, they build up and get harder to resolve.

When I first began to develop a love life, I thought, *Why the hell do we have to talk all the time?* I wasn't used to discussing serious things and I was a bad listener. Talking about problems felt like hard work when we could just pretend they didn't exist or gloss over them by having sex. But after a few years of experience in love, I think talking is what works for the long term.

Exercise: Solve a problem

Choose a small and unimportant problem you have between you. Sit down with a pen, which will serve as a "talking stick," and you have to be holding it if you want to say something. So you can't interrupt each other during the exercise. Try to share the talking stick so both of you get to speak equally.

Begin by saying how each of you feel in that moment. Then you can start talking about the actual problem. Each of you gets to say what you think and feel about the problem, but neither of you is allowed to suggest solutions until each of you has understood the other person's thoughts and feelings.

Once you've exhausted the subject, you should try to find possible solutions and choose a solution that works for both of you and both of you feel happy with. Finish by saying how each of you feels.

Everyone argues sometimes

That you argue or fight doesn't necessarily mean there is anything wrong with the relationship or you should break up. On the contrary, it can be good to be open about having differing opinions. Couples vary in how much they argue. But no matter how laid-back the two of you might be, it's almost impossible to never argue. It's kind of like a law of nature in very close relationships, just like two siblings rarely grow up never having had a fight.

When you argue, you're angry and sad, and you may feel like you're being accused of something. Understandably, at this time it's hard to remember a list from a book, but read my list again after the argument and see how it went! Arguments can be destructive. But they can also be constructive, making the relationship grow and develop in the right direction.

Advice for when you argue

- Take one thing at a time. You might be angry because you don't meet up often enough and you're fed up with your partner's younger siblings. Work out one of the issues first and then the other one. If you talk about both things at the same time, you're not going to get very far.
- Listen. When you're in the middle of an argument, it's easy to feel that the other person is stupid and just throwing accusations at you. But try to take in what they're

saying. Might there be some truth in the complaint that you don't answer texts?

- Don't resort to personal attacks. You might think your partner flirts with other people. In that case you can say so, but don't call them a slut, for example.
- If there are other problems that are making you angry, admit that. You might be angry that your partner arrived half an hour late—but might you be even angrier that you've been dropped from the team you play in?
- Remember that arguing doesn't mean you should break up. It could just as easily mean that you're actually dealing with your problems so the relationship can survive.
- Hours of shouting and crying are perfect fuel for hot and sticky make-up sex once you've worked things out!

You don't own each other

Sometimes people get jealous. Usually it boils down to a problem with yourself rather than the person you're with. You're happy in the relationship but maybe you feel a bit anxious or scared that the person you love will dump you. That will make you suspicious of the people who surround your partner.

If one of you gets jealous, you need to talk about it. What is making the person jealous? Is the relationship really in trouble or is it just something the jealous person has convinced themselves of?

Remember that you don't own each other. Even though you're in a relationship, you still get to make your own decisions. No one can prevent you from going to parties or meeting up with friends. However, you still need to take the jealous person's feelings seriously. Maybe you need to make it even clearer that they are loved.

Sex is not a must

Most people have sex for the first time with someone they're going out with. But you don't have to have sex just because you're going out. In the past, newlyweds were expected to have sex so they could produce heirs to the family fortune. But nowadays, you can have sex without being in love and you can be in love without having sex.

Neither you nor your partner have a responsibility to ensure the other person is sexually satisfied or has their sexual fantasies fulfilled. It's ridiculous to use love to pressure your partner for sex. If you love each other, you won't force the other person into something they don't want to do.

But if both of you want to have sex, there is no reason not to do something you both want.

Be equal together

Relationships are almost never completely equal. There is often something that gives one person a little more power. Imagine one person is a little less in love than their partner. This gives that person the upper hand in the relationship, making it easier for them to be controlling and make decisions. Another factor in the power dynamic is simply who you are when you enter into the relationship. Is one really popular and the other a loner? Is one older than the other? Are they both guys and one is open about his sexuality while the other is still in the closet?

But perhaps the greatest power difference in a relationship comes when one partner is male and the other is female. Boys and men as a group have more power in society and are often encouraged in their male gender role to be more selfish whereas girls and women tend to be encouraged to be selfless and caring.

Inequality in a relationship is bad for both sides. The one with less power risks ending up with low self-esteem. The one with more power risks becoming selfish and irritated with the other person. In all loving relationships it's therefore crucial to make every effort to be equal. And the greatest responsibility for this equality lies with whoever has the upper hand.

Equality is as much about giving as it is taking. If you're with someone who listens when you're down, you should also listen when they're down.

Equality is also about both of you getting to make the decisions. If you went to your cousin's party last weekend, maybe you should go to your partner's friend's party this weekend.

When both of you get just as much out of the relationship and share the power, then you have an equal relationship.

The emotions roller coaster

When I first started discovering love, I overthought things all the time. I thought, *Am I in love now? Right in this second, do I feel like I'm in love? As in love as I was yesterday?*

I recently spoke to my friend Tarek, who told me he did the same thing.

"I was constantly analyzing what I felt. I never relaxed and just let things happen."

Tarek explained that on some days he was incredibly in love, while on others he either felt nothing, felt more stressed about an exam, or felt angry at one of his parents. The feeling of being in love wasn't there.

"That made me nervous. I thought my feelings weren't strong enough, so I had to break it off. But then the next day everything felt good again and I knew I really did want us to be together."

In the movies, couples are completely loved up all the time. But in real life love often comes in waves. Sometimes the love is overwhelming, and sometimes you can hardly feel it. It's up to you to decide whether you want to stay together when the feelings aren't strong, but you can be together without being head over heels in love all the time. Many people who've been together for a long time are more like friends who occasionally discover that they've fallen in love with each other all over again.

Exercise: Gift giving

This game is a good way to show that you like each other and to practice your sensitivity. You and your partner should separately each buy three small gifts. They should be cheap things, like a feather, a Lego toy, a little teddy bear, or some sweets. Use your imagination!

One of you lies on your stomach on the bed with your top off, facedown on the pillow so you can't see anything. The other takes one of the gifts and strokes you with it all over your back and arms. You then have to guess what the gift is. Once you've correctly guessed all three, you get to see the gifts and then you switch places and do the same thing to them.

BREAKING UP

Dan remembers how special he thought Frida was when he met her. She was strong, independent, and a year older than him. Frida was friends with one of Dan's friends. They met at a party and hit it off right away. After that they saw each other every day.

In the second month things began to go downhill.

"She got angry at little things. Once she was furious when I said I'd liked a band for longer than she had. I could tell she was actually angry about something else. She started to get tired of me," says Dan.

Frida wanted to meet up less and less often. Dan thought that if he gave her some space and didn't kick up a fuss, things would return to normal again. He was in love and wanted it to work. One day, when Dan was out in town, Frida called him up.

"She said she wanted to talk. I said I already knew that she wanted to break up. Frida told me I was right. We hung up and then I just sat on a bench and cried," recalls Dan.

Frida came up with various excuses for them not to see each other. It took a week for them to agree to meet for coffee.

"It was good that we did that. She told me it was all over and I needed to hear that, so I didn't go away thinking it could still work out."

Dan feels that everyone around him was supportive when he was upset. But some were better than others in the way they reacted. His best friend just wanted him to party all the time to take his mind off what had happened. But Dan felt he needed time to be sad.

"Funnily enough it was my mom who said the best things. She said Frida was the kind of person who doesn't know what she wants and I would meet someone new eventually."

When I meet Dan, a year has passed since Frida broke up with him. He still gets a knot in his stomach when he thinks about her sometimes, but he feels better now.

"I've accepted that it ended and that I couldn't have done anything to fix things. The way Frida felt about me was out of my control. And I'm not angry either. I don't think you break up with someone to hurt them; it's just that you don't have the same feelings anymore," he says.

Let your feelings out

Being dumped by someone you love can be one of the hardest things to deal with. It can feel like you're going around with a gaping wound day in, day out, and you can feel worthless. In this situation, it's good to let your grief out instead of shutting down your emotions and pretending that you feel fine. Bottling up your feelings just means that they build up and then risk coming out in some other form that may be more difficult to deal with.

Dan is the kind of guy who finds it easy to communicate, so he talked to quite a few people about how he felt. Not everyone is as comfortable with talking as Dan is, but it's good to at least have someone you can work through your thoughts and feelings with. Sometimes people are in the unfortunate position when none of their friends or any of the adults around them understand, so they don't have anyone to talk to. In this case, writing down your thoughts and feelings can make you feel better.

Even though you're down, it can be good to try and find things in the present that are fun or feel good, so you're not completely consumed by the end of your relationship. At some point, you have to rediscover how great life can actually be, despite that special person no longer being around.

If you are dumped

- Don't be mean to the person who dumped you, for example, by saying nasty things about them or spreading rumors. Your ex can't control their emotions and they're probably also sad that it ended.
- Demand clarity. If it's over, the person needs to tell it to you straight, so you know and can move on.
- When things are tough, you'll feel better after a good cry.

Don't want to hurt anyone

Jamal laughs and jokes a lot and finds it easy talking to people he doesn't know. He often hangs out at the youth club near where he lives and that was where he met his former girlfriend Jenny.

To start with he really liked Jenny, and their relationship worked well. But over time Jamal's feelings faded, and he no longer wanted to go out with her. The problem was that he felt he couldn't break it off.

"You could see that she was so in love with me. She was a year or so younger than me and I think she looked up to me a little. I knew she would be really upset if I ended it," says Jamal.

And so he hatched a plan to avoid hurting his girlfriend. He would make sure Jenny dumped him instead. Jamal changed the way he behaved. He began to arrive late every time they arranged to meet, and he didn't hang out with her as much. Instead he spent almost all of his time with his friends.

But the plan didn't work. His girlfriend stayed with him.

"It was hard work seeing her take all this shit even though it upset her. She was too much in love to end things. I knew that what I'd done was not cool," says Jamal.

Finally Jamal decided to talk to Jenny. He said he wasn't in love with her and she cried. It was hard, but afterward Jamal felt relieved that it was finally over.

Make the best of it

Jamal now thinks he handled the breakup badly and feels it would have been kinder to end things early on, as soon as he knew he was no longer in love. The way he dragged it out hardly made Jenny feel better, and it didn't drive her to break up with him, as he'd thought it would.

Naturally, hurting someone feels terrible, but sometimes you can't avoid it. In this case it's best to dump the other person in a way that allows them to move on as quickly as possible. Tell them clearly that it's over. Then listen to what your ex has to say and let them cry, even if it makes you feel uncomfortable. If your ex has questions, answer them.

People who are dumped sometimes think there's something wrong with them. They may think, *You wanted us to be together a few weeks ago, so why not now?* Your ex may think you're dumping them because they've changed for the worse somehow. But the fact that you're calling time on the relationship may well have nothing to do with your ex's personality; it may just be that your feelings have changed. It's important that you help your ex ditch any thoughts that they are unattractive, bad in bed, or anything else.

If you break it off

- Don't dump someone by just disappearing or by phone, email, text, letter, messenger, telegram, or smoke signals. Talk face-to-face and give the conversation the time it needs.
- End it in a place where you can talk privately.
- Be clear that it's really over.

R E S P E C T

SHOW RESPECT

If you want to be good at love and sex, you also have to be respectful. Everyone has been disrespected at some point, so we all know how it feels. When someone is disrespectful, they're showing that they see themselves as better than others and therefore feel they have the right to abuse people.

All relationships between two people need respect. When someone is disrespectful, we close up. Why would anyone share their deepest secrets with someone who shows no respect? To really get to know and understand someone, you have to be respectful. This is true in a relationship with someone you're going out with, someone you're sleeping with, or any other kind of relationship.

You benefit from being respectful because it inclines other people to be more honest and open. At the same time, the world is a little more relaxed when you behave well toward others.

If you want to be respectful, all you usually have to do is treat others the way you would like to be treated. But when it comes to girls, things are slightly different.

Because we live in a society where girls as a group have less power, it's also more common for girls to encounter a lack of respect. I'll be describing some typical ways that girls are disrespected in everyday life and give you techniques for turning the situations around as a guy.

It's important as a guy to distance yourself from and take a stand against the disrespecting of girls. Disrespect has been around for thousands of years, and it's up to us as young people to decide whether it's going to live on or disappear.

This is what teenage girls experience in one year at high school:

- 77 percent hear demeaning comments about being a girl
- 71 percent are rated on their attractiveness
- 52 percent are given sexual looks
- 37 percent are called a whore or something similar
- 27 percent are groped
- 26 percent are pressured for sex
- 25 percent have sexual rumors spread about them
- 0.2 percent are raped

> Together we guys can get these
> figures down to zero.*

GUYS IN A GROUP

Almost every guy I've met has been really clued in when I've spoken to them in a room one-on-one. It makes me wonder how there can be such a lack of respect when there are so many aware guys around.

But sometimes people change when they're with their friends. You may not even notice it yourself, but it's quite common for guys to be a bit more disrespectful when others are watching.

In my local newspaper awhile back, I read an interview with a guy who was sitting with his group of buddies. He said he controlled his sister and beat her. He also said he thought some girls were whores.

This is the kind of guy that some adults get angry about and refer to as a "pig." But I thought this must just be a facade, not the real him.

And so it was that in the next edition of the local newspaper, he was interviewed again. This time he was on his own, without his friends. He had asked to be interviewed again, because his family had been disappointed in him. In a new article he admitted he had lied; he didn't control his sister in any way and certainly didn't beat her. And he apologized for saying that girls were whores.

---

*Source: Eva Witkowska, *Sexual Harassment in Schools: Prevalence, Structure and Perceptions* (Stockholm: Arbetslivsinstitutet [National Institute for Working Life], 2005), 26.

"I'm ashamed and I'm sorry; I'm really not that guy," he said. When the journalist asked him why he had said all these things, he replied: "That's what happens when you're with your friends."

The unusual thing about this story is that the guy ended up in the newspaper. But otherwise, I think he's like most people. When the mask drops, there's a pretty good person behind it.

Respect technique #1: Respect yourself

As a guy you sometimes have to choose between being kind to others or gaining street cred from your friends. It's a tough choice, because no one wants to look like a wuss. But if you respect yourself, you don't pretend to be a worse person than you actually are. It's a kind of crime against yourself to be good deep down but shout things at girls, for example, in front of your friends. Above all, it's no comfort to the girl if you're good deep down but not showing it.

Behave in a way that you can be proud of. If you're ever expected to be disrespectful, say what you think instead. Many people will think it's brave of you to say no, even if they don't say so out loud. Once you've said what you think a few times, your friends will get used to it and it won't be a big thing anymore.

It's been scientifically proven that we are affected by being in a group. Researcher Solomon Asch conducted an experiment involving young men. A test subject went into a classroom with other young men who were secretly the researcher's assistants. The group had to answer some simple questions.

The test subject correctly answered the questions as long as the rest of the group did the same. But when the assistants began giving incorrect answers, the test subject tended to do the same as the rest of the group, despite the right answer being obvious.

Fully 75 percent of the test subjects gave incorrect answers. So most people find it more difficult to go against group pressure than to say something they know is wrong.

GROPING

It was when I started having female friends that I began to understand how much girls plan their lives around the fear of rapists. Instead of relaxing when there was a party, my female friends would often plan in advance how they were going to get home and who would keep them company. Some places were almost no-go areas at night. Sometimes they would rather take a long detour than use the short route through a park. And when they walked home through an unfamiliar area, they would call me and talk all the way. That way, if a rapist attacked them, I would know and could quickly call the police.

Why were they so scared? I couldn't understand it. Rape outdoors is extremely uncommon. There's a greater risk of being robbed or assaulted. And yet my female friends were so afraid that it restricted their ability to have fun.

When I asked them about it, my female friends said that the fear had been established early on and that a lot of guys had helped to create their fear. They talked about guys who groped them and catcalled them and commented on their appearance in disrespectful ways as they walked past. And no other guys had told them to stop. This had taught my female friends that they didn't have power over their own bodies, and so they became scared of what might happen to them if they encountered a guy they didn't know when they were alone. What many guys saw as a joke, the girls experienced as terror.

Respect technique #2: Don't cross other people's boundaries

No one is allowed to touch you against your will or force you to have sex, because only you can decide such matters regarding your body. It's important that other people respect your ownership of your body, and it's also important for you to respect other people's bodies. You do this by not groping, rating physical appearance, or calling out things like "Nice ass!" when a girl walks by.

If you want to make contact with a girl because you're interested, any other way is better than demeaning her!

If a friend gropes or verbally harasses a girl, you can stand up for her by asking your friend some questions. "Why did you do that?" "How do you think she feels when you do that?" "Would you want people to do that to your sister?" Asking questions means that your friend has to think, in which case you might win him over to your side.

Groping, unwanted sexual looks, comments such as slut or fag, or spreading sexual rumors count as sexual harassment and are against the law. Both guys and girls can experience sexual harassment. The school is responsible for ensuring that it stops.

The greatest risk of being groped at school is in these places:*

1. The corridor
2. By the lockers
3. The classroom
4. The schoolyard
5. The break room
6. The gym
7. Near the restrooms

SLUTTINESS

Many of the girls I talk to explain that they have to walk a tightrope when it comes to sexuality. If a girl has never kissed anyone and doesn't have any sexy outfits, she's labeled as boring, and no guy will

---

*Source: Christina Osbeck, Ann-Sofie Holm, and Inga Wernersson, *Kränkningar i skolan : förekomst, former och sammanhang* [*Violations in School: Occurrence, Forms and Contexts*] (Gothenburg: Gothenburg University, 2003), 99.

be interested in her. So to get attention, she has to at least be slightly sexy and slightly available. The problem is that she mustn't be too available or too sexy, because then she's branded a slut.

"At break time in my school, some guys talk about girls, particularly girls in eighth grade, who they've been with. They loudly tell everyone what they did with the girl, and they do it in a demeaning way, as if they think the girls are cheap. One guy pressured a girl in school to have anal sex. Then he badmouthed her in front of the whole school because she'd gone along with it," recalls Linnea.

The guys that Linnea is talking about think it's OK that they're having sex and boasting about what they've done. At the same time, they think the girls shouldn't do it or they should feel ashamed if they do.

Girls have the same feelings in their body as guys do, and so it should be just as OK for a girl to be horny as it is for a guy. It's disrespectful to judge people by different standards, and that's exactly what you're doing if you think a guy can boast while a girl should be ashamed even though both have done exactly the same thing.

> Half of girls in their first year of high school would like to have more sexual experiences than they actually have.*

*Source: Boris Klanger, Tanja Tydén, and Leena Ruusuvaara, "Sexual Behavior Among Adolescents in Uppsala, Sweden," *Journal of Adolescent Health* 14, no. 6 (September 1993): 468–74.

Anna is another girl I spoke to. When she was in junior high, she wasn't popular and didn't have sex. She says she really wanted to do it and get to see what it felt like. But the rules that are set around girls' sexuality stopped her.

"All the girls said it was slutty to have sex for the first time with someone who wasn't your boyfriend. That meant I couldn't have sex, because I didn't have a boyfriend. I would actually have been happy to have sex with a classmate, but losing your virginity to a classmate was a no-no; only a slut would do that," says Anna.

The risk of being labeled a slut is an obstacle for girls who want to explore their sexuality, but it also makes it more difficult for guys to get to sleep with girls.

Respect technique #3: Stop spreading sexual rumors

If you've heard that a girl has slept with a lot of guys, don't call her a slut. If she has slept with lots of people, so what? It's her body, and it's up to her what she does with it. No one else has the right to judge her. And all the things people say may not be true.

When someone is called a slut, you can show respect by not spreading rumors and by not agreeing that the girl is a slut.

If you yourself have made out or had sex with a girl, you also have a responsibility not to gossip about her afterward. Simply don't tell people the details of what you did and didn't do. It's something good that happened between the two of you. Don't risk getting half the school involved, as they could destroy the whole experience for you.

If you hear a male friend calling a girl a slut, ask some questions that will make him think. "Girls get just as horny as guys, so why should girls be ashamed of it, but not guys?" or "What business is it of other people how much sex a girl has?" or "If girls aren't allowed to have sex, how can guys ever have sex with girls?"

HONOR

When Farman was a few years younger than he is now, he used to control and make decisions for his sisters. For example, he decided that they couldn't go to any clubs. He thought many girls were slutty and didn't want other guys to think the same thing about his own sisters. Farman also thought his honor was tied up with his sisters' sexuality. If his sisters went to parties and made out, Farman would lose face.

One day his parents found a text message from a guy on his big sister's phone. They beat her and demanded to know who the guy was. They were afraid that he was her boyfriend. But the sister said they were just friends.

Farman went out with some friends and tracked the guy down. The guy repeated what the sister had said: they went to the same school and were friends. Farman threatened the guy and told him not to contact his sister again.

"At the time, I was in high school and had several friends who were girls. They would text me and it was all perfectly normal. But when my sister got a text, I saw it differently," says Farman.

Eventually, the notion of honor came back to bite Farman. It was when he got a girlfriend. The girl's family didn't want her to date anyone. They had to meet in secret and when they were discovered, Farman was threatened by his girlfriend's brother.

"That's when I began to think, *Why should someone else decide how I should feel and what I do?*"

After that, Farman talked to his family and a lot changed. Today, Farman thinks differently about his sisters and girls in general, and he's glad about that. Now he can talk openly with his sisters, and they don't have to keep things secret. He also no longer needs to worry about losing face in front of his friends, because it's no longer an issue. He no longer feels that how his sisters are living their lives has anything to do with his honor.

> Guys can also be subjected to honor-based oppression; for example if they fall in love with another guy or with the "wrong" girl or if, in some other way, they step outside the family's expectations about how to live.

Honor as a concept runs through the whole of society and isn't necessarily tied to the country you were born in or your religion. When I was in junior high, guys would—half jokingly and half seriously—warn other guys to stay away from their sister. That's a milder form of honor-based behavior.

Respect technique #4: Don't control other people

Don't stand in the way of a girl who wants to make her own decisions about love and sex. Also don't snitch if you see a girl with a guy or at a party if you know that the girl's family doesn't allow it. It's the girl's life and she has a right to live it however she wants.

You also have the right to live without being forced to keep control over others. Sometimes families try to force a son to control a sister, even though he doesn't want to. In this case, it's best to talk to your sister. Maybe you can both find a way to resolve the problem. In the best case, you can speak to your sister and then talk to your family. Then the family can find a solution, such as maintaining a facade for the relatives, while letting everyone be free within the family.

Talk to an adult who can give you support—for example, someone trustworthy and wise at school or at a youth center.

If it feels wrong to you that your sister has a love life or a sex life, maybe you need to change your attitude toward girls. If you don't see girls as sluts, no one will be able to diss you by commenting on your sister.

SPACE

Many girls I've talked to have mentioned that guys as a group take up much more space than girls. Josefin names a typical example from the club she's actively involved in.

"When we have meetings, they're really long, because all the guys want to speak in front of the group. Even when everything there is to say has been said, the guys want to carry on talking. They repeat what each other has said but in different words. It feels like they think the important thing isn't to say something new, just to say something," explains Josefin.

There are also girls in the club. But according to Josefin, the girls don't talk as much.

"Sometimes I have something to say that no one has thought of, but I keep quiet. The meetings end up so long because the guys talk so much, so I think it's best not to make things longer by speaking up.

But after the meeting I'm sometimes angry at myself for not saying what I thought," says Josefin.

Many girls have said they think there are different standards for girls and boys when it comes to taking up space. They feel that boys are allowed to get away with things whereas girls can't afford to make mistakes; they have to be at the top of their game all the time. Aida gives an example.

"If we're playing soccer and a boy passes the ball to another boy and he loses it, nothing happens. But if a boy passes to a girl and she loses the ball, the other boys moan 'Why did you pass to a girl!' The boys get more chances to make mistakes and practice until they get better," says Aida.

Respect technique #5: Listen and give space

Listen when others are talking. Listening is not just about letting the sound from the other person's mouth go in through your ears. It's about looking at the person and not rustling paper when the person is speaking, for example. If there's something you want to add or something you think is wrong, you can have your say once the other person has finished speaking. Don't interrupt.

On average, guys take up around two-thirds of classroom time, while girls take up one-third of the time.*

*Source: Moa Elf Karlén and Johanna Palmström, *Ta betalt! : en feministisk överlevnadsguide* [*Get Paid!: A Feminist Survival Guide*] (Stockholm: Rabén & Sjögren, 2004), 10–12.

Some people don't tend to put themselves forward, despite maybe having a lot to say. This is particularly common among girls, who are brought up to be quiet. You can help a person to make themselves heard by inviting them to speak. All you have to do is ask a question like "What do you think?"

Don't punish a person, for example, by laughing, if they get a question wrong. That might make them hesitant about occupying the space again.

Listening and including people can be done in different ways depending on the context. When you're talking you can ask a question, when you're playing soccer you can pass the ball. What other ways are there to listen and include people in your everyday life?

CHORES

When I meet women in early adulthood, around the age of twenty, they sometimes tell me they're unhappy about the fact that their boyfriends don't do any housework. This might seem like a minor issue, but when I speak to the girls themselves, it's clearly a big problem.

"Love might not survive if you have to nag a guy about these things all the time. I'm actually thinking about dumping my boyfriend if he doesn't get his act together soon," one girl told me at a party.

The problem of guys not doing certain types of work starts early. Often parents expect different things from sons and daughters. The daughters are required to help out in the home. The sons are more likely to get away with not helping.

The same thing sometimes also happens in schools, with teachers using girls to keep the class and the classroom in order. Boys tend not to have the same responsibility.

When you're a teenager, this is a problem you might not even notice. But if you're a guy who likes girls and you want to live with a girl when you're older, you're guaranteed to have problems if you don't learn how to handle chores such as doing the dishes and the like.

When you're an adult, you'll probably see this as the most important piece of advice in the whole book for guys who want to live happily with girls.

Respect technique #6: Share chores equally

Girls are not servants or slaves who should clean and cook for guys. If you respect the equal value of women and men, you should share the chores equally.

> The vast majority of guys think you should take equal responsibility, whatever your gender. Ninety-two percent of young men polled in Sweden want to share equal responsibility for chores in the home and for the children when they have a family.*

---

*Source: The Swedish Agency for Youth and Civil Society, *Unga Med Attityd 2013* [*Young with Attitude 2013*] (Stockhom: The Swedish Agency for Youth and Civil Society, 2013), 78.

If you have a sister and you notice your parents giving your sister more chores, you can ask them to give you the same amount to do. If that doesn't work, help your sister. You could alternate, so that every other time your parents tell your sister to empty the dishwasher, you can say "No, I'll do it instead,"

The same applies in other situations. Maybe your class is on a school trip and you're staying at a youth hostel. On the last day, you have to make sure the cabin is clean. Typically in such situations, suddenly all the guys disappear and the girls are left to do all the cleaning themselves. Don't be one of those guys. Volunteer to help with the work without anyone having to tell you.

These are the respect techniques:

1. Respect yourself.
2. Don't cross other people's boundaries.
3. Stop spreading rumors.
4. Don't control other people.
5. Listen and give space.
6. Share chores equally.

5

SEX: THE BASICS

THE IMAGE OF SEX

Turn on the TV and compare the sex in a few TV series or films. You'll notice that the sex is mostly depicted in the same way. There's a man and a woman. They kiss each other as they undress. Then they insert the penis into the vagina and hump away. Ten seconds later both have climaxed and they lie next to each other looking happy.

The sex is the same in the biology textbooks. They often say things like "When the penis is erect, it can be inserted into the vagina." Sex is described as something that you do to have children, even though people mostly have sex for pleasure.

Society basically has a picture of what sex should look like, and it's supposed to be a dick in a vagina, representing sexual intercourse between a girl and a guy. Sex and intercourse tend to be portrayed as the same thing, which is not true. Intercourse is one of many different types of sex. There are many ways a guy and a girl can have sex other than sexual intercourse. Plus guys may want to sleep with guys and girls may want to sleep with girls.

Because the same image of sex is repeated over and over, you might get a sense that the image is the "right way" to do it. And everyone wants to do the right thing. This image of sex therefore influences the way we choose to have sex. Many guys and girls follow the ideal even though they might get more pleasure from doing it a different way.

I think it's a shame to close the door on the diverse range of sex that's actually available. Particularly if you plan on having sex for your entire life, doing the same thing every time might get a little repetitive.

MAKING OUT

It is sometimes hard to decide where the boundary is between "sex" and everything else. After all, you can get pleasure and reach orgasm without even taking your clothes off. Where is the line for what counts as sex? That's something you have to decide.

In this book, "making out" means everything you can do without directly touching naked genitals. But make sure you have the other person's permission before moving beyond kissing.

Take your time to explore the other person's smell, taste, warmth, and body while making out! Enjoy the feelings you get when the other person explores you, and there's no end to the ways you can do it. Experiment by doing things that excite you. Pay attention to each other's body language so neither of you goes farther than the other one wants to. Often, you'll see it feels like enough just to be kissing and holding each other.

Sometimes people who have begun having sex completely forget about making out, not least because sex can seem like it would always be more desirable. But sometimes you're not up for sex and you just want to make out, and then it's absolutely the desirable option. Even if you want to have sex, making out is a great way to start. It works up the emotions and creates an exciting atmosphere that makes your body more sensitive when you then have sex.

Taking off a bra

If you're making out with a girl who's wearing a bra you want to take off, it can sometimes be easiest to ask her to unclip it so you can remove it. But if you want to unclip it yourself and you're not completely sure what to do, the best thing is for her to sit up with her back to you. That way you'll be able to see the clasp as you undo it. While you're working away, kiss her on the neck and stroke her back to make the bra removal a sensual part of making out.

A few ways to make out

- Kiss each other. Again. And again.
- Press your bodies against each other. It's a nice sensation and it's exciting to feel the other person's heat against your body.
- If both of you want, making out can involve more than kissing. Run your hands over the other person's clothes. And don't just focus on the chest, genitals, and butt. Try other places, like the arms and back.
- You can stroke the face. Try doing it very lightly with one or more fingertips, running them over the eyebrows, the cheeks, and the lips, for example.
- Put a hand under the person's shirt and stroke the stomach and waist.
- Suck on parts of the neck and shoulders. If you suck too hard, you can cause a hickey, which not everyone likes. Hickeys are caused by burst blood vessels and they can last a few days before they disappear.
- Wrestling or tickling. Some people like to play around. Play can release any performance anxiety and make things feel less tense.
- Lick or suck on the ear. Start gently, for example, by licking the earlobe a little. You can also suck on the earlobe, but take it easy. If you go in too hard, it can cause unpleasant shivers.

- Rub your genitals against each other through your clothes. You can also rub genitals in the sex positions presented later in the book. It's exciting because it makes you imagine what it would be like to do these things naked....
- Touch the other person's genitals outside their clothes.
- Touch the ass, for example starting at the top of the butt crack and moving downward, or caress the butt cheeks.
- Take off the person's top and stroke them down the spine.
- Taking each other's clothes off can be exciting. Draw out the excitement by not taking everything off at once. Make out for a while, then take off their shirt. Make out some more. Then take off their pants. Slowly, you get access to more skin.
- You can stroke, lick, and suck the nipples and the area around them. Go gently as both girls and guys can find it painful if you're too heavy-handed. Remember that there is more to the chest and breasts than just the nipples.
- Touch the genitals outside the underwear. If it's a girl and you notice that her panties are wet, you can rub that spot with a finger. If it's a guy, you can take hold of his erection outside his boxers.
- Lick the armpits. It might tickle, but it can also feel great.
- If you bite each other gently it can feel like a painless caress.
- Run your hand over the inner thighs with long, slow strokes. You can also kiss and suck this area.

- Put an ice cube between your lips and run it over the other person's body like a cold caress. It might not be something to do the first time you make out with someone, but many people find that the cold gives a wonderful burning sensation.
- Say sexy things. For example, you can say what you want to do to each other.
- Place your mouth against your partner's underwear and breathe warm, moist air onto the genitals. Caress the genitals outside the underwear with your nose and lips. Kiss and suck the underwear.

FIRST TIME

One day in high school after gym, one of the guys in my class undressed in the locker room. His skin was marked with little hickeys, spread all over his body like the spots on a Dalmatian. He took his towel and strode proudly into the shower while we all looked on in wonder.

He'd done it. What all the guys talked about. But there was a big difference between the usual banter and this. The guys in school boasted a lot, but we all understood that it was all mostly lies. This guy had proof.

I felt like I didn't want to get undressed and go into the shower. My body had no hickeys, and I felt like a failure. We guys egged each other on, and it felt like we had a competition going to have sex as soon as possible.

Half of guys have not had sex by the age of seventeen,
and it's the same for girls.*

The male gender role creates the expectation that a guy should be able to get sex. That's why having sex often seems to gain you higher status among your friends. And the more people you have sex with, the more recognition you get for it.

This part of the male gender role is fine for those who enjoy having sex with different people and for guys who are really outgoing. But not all guys are interested in sex. And not everyone enjoys having sex with lots of different people. I talked to Nils about this—he has sex with guys.

"After one night stands I think, *Why did I do that?* It's not even that enjoyable. Often when I have one-night stands, I actually want to just kiss and sleep together. Sex feels best when I'm going out with someone," says Nils.

Work out what you want to do about sex. If you want to sleep around, do so. But do it because you enjoy it, not to raise your status with your friends.

Don't rush it

The first chance I got to have sex, I was invited back to the home of a person I hung out with, whose parents were away. On the one hand I

---

*Source: National Center for Health Statistics, "Key Statistics from the National Survey of Family Growth," Centers for Disease Control and Prevention, June 23, 2017, www.cdc.gov/nchs/nsfg/key_statistics/d.htm.

wanted to do it. I wasn't particularly popular and being one of the first in the class to have sex would give me an ego boost.

But at the same time, the feeling in my gut was all wrong. I felt anxious and nervous. It really didn't feel like a fun thing to do. In my imagination sex was cool, but in reality it was terrifying. So I said no. But it wasn't something I was proud of or told people about; I kept that no to myself.

The age at which you can legally consent to have sex varies by state in the U.S., but the most common (and lowest age) is sixteen. This law is in place to protect children and young people from assault by adults. But there are close-in-age exemptions for teenagers, so you won't be in trouble with the law as long as you are roughly the same age.

Two years later I got another chance, and this time I took it. It was at a party, I'd had a bit to drink, but I wasn't completely drunk. We made out a little on the sofa and then we sneaked off to a bedroom. The sex was giggly. I never thought sex could be giggly, but this sex was. I thought it was fun and exciting. It felt quite pleasurable, but not nearly as pleasurable as I thought it would. What I enjoyed most was having another person so close and so naked.

I left the party walking on air. It was like I'd opened a secret door into another world. And I'd only caught a glimpse of that world; there was an awful lot more to explore.

I felt more grown-up.

But having sex for the first time doesn't always go the way you thought it would. When I talk to guys about their first time, I hear stories both happy and sad. Ahmed tells his story: "I was probably too young. There'd been so much talk about doing it, so when I got my chance I felt I had to take it. But the sex itself was terrible. It still makes me anxious when I think about it. It was really not nice, and she thought the same. I forced my way through it and then vowed never to have sex again. I stuck to that for a few years," says Ahmed.

How you know you're ready

- You're doing it for your own sake, not for status or cred from others.
- It feels exciting.
- The person you're going to do it with feels like someone you want to have sex with. You feel comfortable and horny with her or him.
- You have experience of making out or have at least kissed or touched someone before. If you don't have any experience, you might want to take things slower. Make out today, have sex tomorrow?
- You have a good feeling in your stomach.

Often when guys talk about their bad introduction to sex, I think it sounds like they actually weren't ready to do it. I'm glad, therefore, that I didn't pressure myself into taking the first chance that came my way and instead waited until I felt more comfortable about having sex.

You decide when the right time is for you. Put the brakes on if it feels bad. And if it feels good, go with it!

Many first times

The initiation into sex is sometimes called losing your virginity. Personally, I don't use the word *virginity* because I don't believe you lose anything when you have sex, particularly not any kind of virginal innocence. What you get is an experience and an encounter with another person.

I also don't like the idea of virginity because you can only lose it once. It's all bound up with an idealized image of sex. Because sexual intercourse is the only thing that counts as "real" sex, you can only have sex for the first time once. But in my view, there are many different kinds of sex, and so there are also many occasions when you do something for the first time. The first time with someone you love. The first time outdoors. The first time you have oral sex. The first time you have sexual intercourse. The first time you both have an orgasm. There are endless first times.

That's why I think we shouldn't place too much emphasis on the very first time. If you didn't think it went well, it might go better the next time you do something for the first time.

In a survey, 50 percent of guys and girls said their first sexual intercourse encounter was good. When asked what they thought about their most recent intercourse, 90 percent felt it was good. Basically, sex gets better once you've had some practice.*

Sometimes guys have asked me if I have any tips for the very first time. By definition, you have no experience at this point and might not know what you're supposed to be doing in that moment. We all work differently when it comes to sex, but by adhering to the advice that follows and talking with your partner about what they like, you'll have a better time.

How to make your first time a good time

- Make out a lot! Some guys seem to think you should just take off your clothes and get down to it. But making out before sex is the key to having a pleasurable time together and not making it feel awkward. Take your time making out and gradually build up to the sex.

---

*Source: Elisabet Häggström-Nordin, Ulf Hanson, Tanja Tydén, "Associations between Pornography Consumption and Sexual Practices among Adolescents in Sweden," *International Journal of STD and AIDS* 16, no. 2 (February 2005): 102–7.

- Lower your expectations. It's not going to be the best sex of your life. It may not be all that enjoyable and the two of you may only keep going for a short while. If you go in with the attitude that it's going to be an earth-shattering experience, there's every chance you'll be disappointed. See it for what it is, your first step into a sex life.

- Don't try doing advanced stuff the first time you have sex. Instead, focus on getting to know the other person's body, how it feels, and what it feels like when your body is explored. It would be best not to have sexual intercourse the very first time you or your partner have sex. It can easily go wrong if the participants are a little nervous.

- You don't need to come. Nerves make it hard to reach orgasm, and in such a situation there's no point trying to force the issue. Focus instead on exploring what gives the other person pleasure.

LOSING YOUR HARD-ON

I remember once talking to a male friend about losing your hard-on. He said all guys had lost their erection at some time or other.

"Particularly when you're drunk, then it can be impossible to get it up," he said.

I didn't recognize this at all, as I'd never not been able to get a hard-on. But just a few weeks later, I went to a party and got drunk. I hooked up with a person and went home with them. We undressed . . . and then I couldn't get it up!

But there was no drama involved.

"I'm clearly too drunk. I think I need to sleep," I said. And so we slept instead.

> Many guys find their erection comes and goes during sex. You can have sex and enjoy it without having an erection. A quarter of guys can reach orgasm without an erection.*

There are many reasons for not getting an erection. When you're young, it's not about being impotent. It's more likely to be a case of nerves, because you really want it to go well. Or maybe you're not used to sex and it feels a bit scary—that can kill a hard-on. Many people also drink alcohol to give them the courage to have sex, and doing so can also affect your erection.

You really don't need to worry about losing your hard-on. It's something all guys experience sooner or later.

If you often lose your erection

- Take the sex more slowly, so you get a chance to build up your feelings.

---

*Source: Shere Hite, *The Hite Report on Male Sexuality* (New York: Knopf, 1981), 1097–99.

- Lower your demands on yourself. Maybe you can just forget the erection and have sex without it?
- Be honest with yourself. Is this a person you're really interested in? Do you really feel comfortable with having sex? Or are you forcing yourself into sex?
- Maybe there are other things in your life that are distracting you. For example, there might be problems at home or other things you need to resolve to feel good and get an erection more easily.
- If you drink or take drugs or are tired, you can try not drinking, not taking drugs, or getting some rest.
- Book an appointment to discuss the issue with your doctor. They can help you work out why you often lose your erection.

YES AND NO

When you have sex, you have a responsibility to read the signals from the other person. When I make out with or sleep with someone, I always keep an eye out for signals. They can mean the person either likes or doesn't like what I'm doing. If the person seems to like something I'm doing, I can do more of the same because I know they're enjoying it. By listening to the signals, I can also try new things and see what my partner thinks about them. The signals essentially provide you with a compass to navigate your way through the sex. If I follow the signals, I know my partner is having a good time.

When you have sex, it's always important to get positive signals from the other person, because they mean both that the person is enjoying it and that the person wants to do what you're doing. Listening to the signals shows that I respect my partner's boundaries. The person I'm sleeping with can feel comfortable and relaxed with me. By listening to signals, you're ensuring that you're having sex on both people's terms and both of you are having a good time.

"No" signals

Reading the "yes" signals is all very well, but you also need to keep an eye out for "no" signals at the same time. If, for example, you unbutton someone's trousers and get a "no" signal, that can mean three different things. Either the person thinks things are going too fast and you should slow down and leave the trousers till later. Or the person means they really don't want you to take their trousers off, either now or later, but want to continue making out. But it can also mean the person has no desire to continue making out at all, in which case you should stop immediately.

When you get a "no" signal, it's best to stop and ask the person what they want. Otherwise there's a risk that you'll misunderstand and continue making out, for example, even though the no was a no to everything.

Once when I slept with a person, it felt like things were going really well, but then I received a "no" signal. I wasn't pleased, but I broke off the sex and lay back on the bed.

"Why did you stop?" my partner asked.

"What do you mean? You wanted us to stop, didn't you?" I replied.

"No, I just wanted us to do it a different way."

"Yes" signals you should look out for

They . . .

- say yes,
- look like they're enjoying it,
- make sounds of arousal,
- press themselves against you,
- caress you,
- kiss you,
- help you take off their clothes,
- take the initiative when you do things,
- appear to feel comfortable,
- hold you, or
- giggle, laugh, or smile.

"No" signals you should look out for

They . . .

- say no,
- look like they're in pain,
- appear to have fallen asleep,
- are too drunk or drugged to have control over the situation,

- are completely silent,
- lie with their arms or hands between you,
- seem uncertain or afraid,
- don't kiss you back,
- stiffen up,
- lie still, or
- don't send out any "yes" signals. This is perhaps the most common "no" signal!

Wordless communication is sometimes difficult to interpret and can lead to misunderstandings, like in this case. That's why it's good to ask! "Does it feel good?" "What do you want me to do?" "Would you like me to . . . ?" "Would you like us to take it slower?" "Do you want us to stop?"

No exceptions

Rape is when someone has sex with another person even though that person is sending out "no" signals or is not sending out any "yes" signals. The word *no* doesn't specifically have to be said for it to be rape and it also doesn't have to involve violence.

The media often paint rapists as evil men who lurk in the bushes in an unlit park. But the reality is very different. Rapes mostly take place indoors, and often the rapist is someone in the victim's circle, such as a boyfriend.

Many rapists find it hard to understand that what they did to someone was rape. They didn't lurk in any bushes in an unlit park and they're just ordinary guys, not monsters.

If you don't want to be an ordinary guy who subjects someone to rape, it's important to understand that there are no exceptions in sex. It makes no difference whether you're horny or drunk or together or the other person is skimpily dressed, promised to have sex, or started having sex but then changed their mind. As soon as you get a "no" signal or no longer get "yes" signals, you have to stop.

The laws about consent vary by state in the U.S., but there are three things you will always need to consider:*

- Affirmative Consent: Did the person express overt actions or words indicating agreement for sexual acts?
- Freely Given Consent: Was the consent offered of the person's own free will, without being induced by fraud, coercion, violence, or threat of violence?
- Capacity to Consent: Did the individual have the capacity, or legal ability, to consent?

Pressuring someone into sex

Sexual pressure is a less talked about concept than rape, despite it probably being more common. Sexual pressure is when you pressure someone until they do what you want.

---

*Source: Rape, Abuse & Incest National Network, "Legal Role of Consent," https://www.rainn .org/articles/legal-role-consent.

I interview Markus, a guy who pressured girls into sex a few years ago and now regrets what he did.

"Pressuring someone into sex is about not respecting the other person's boundaries. As I see it there are two types of sexual pressure. One type is where you keep nagging, going 'Come on, come on' all the time. That's not what I did. Instead I put the pressure on with my body," says Markus.

Markus's pressure involved slowly stretching the other person's boundaries. He would put his hand on a girl's thigh. When she moved his hand away, he would put it back. He continued to put it back until she eventually gave up.

Then he had sex with her.

"It wasn't something she wanted to do, but she didn't say no nor did she seem to feel bad about it. It was something she did just to get rid of me," explained Markus.

Pressuring someone into sex is thus a form of assault. Guys and girls both apply sexual pressure. When girls do it, they sometimes play the gay card. They might say "Come on, you're not gay, are you? Sleep with me, then" or threaten to spread a rumor that the guy turned down sex and therefore must be gay.

Pressure in a relationship

Another kind of pressure is emotional blackmail. This form of pressure happens mostly in loving relationships and involves one person using emotions to pressure the other person into sex.

Emotional blackmail typically involves a person saying things like "If you really loved me you would . . ." or "My last girlfriend [or boyfriend] used to . . ." Getting angry or upset because the other person doesn't want to have sex is also emotional blackmail. This pressure is based on making the person you're with feel bad and guilting them into having sex or doing certain things in bed.

Don't use emotional blackmail on someone you like—it shows a complete lack of respect. If you experience it yourself, remember that you don't have a duty to sleep with someone just because you're together. Being in love doesn't mean you agree to everything.

Set boundaries

"Guys always want to have sex!" says a guy in a school I visit. His friends laugh and nod.

"So does that mean you'd sleep with absolutely anyone?" I ask.

"No, maybe not absolutely anyone," he replies.

According to the male gender role, guys are supposed to always be horny, and many guys therefore pretend that they would sleep with anyone just to get some sex. But guys have feelings, thoughts, and tastes just like girls. Sometimes you're tired, sad, or angry and so you don't feel horny. Sometimes you think it would be more interesting to talk and get to know each other instead of having sex.

Not everyone gets you aroused, and not every kind of sex is tempting. Sometimes you may not be interested in sex at all.

As a guy, having sex might get you status and validation from others. It can therefore feel like you have to say yes to any sex that's offered. But you shouldn't go through with sex if you don't have a good gut feeling about it. Your gut feeling is the feeling you have in your body, expressed in ways such as horniness, excitement, uncertainty, or fear. Sometimes your thoughts and your gut feeling might be at odds with each other. For example you might think *This person is attractive, so I should sleep with them*, whereas your gut says no. Listen to your gut feeling and always say no if it doesn't feel good.

In this book, you'll learn various techniques for having sex. But one condition for all of them is that you are able to set your own boundaries and not force yourself into things you don't actually want to do. At the same time, you must also listen to the other person's signals and always take them seriously.

6
STRAIGHT OR GAY?

WHO DO I LIKE?

It's possible that you might be wondering who you like. Girls? Guys? Both? Maybe you think you know exactly how you feel, until you meet someone you find attractive or you have a sex dream that turns your image of yourself upside down.

Only you know what you like. No one else can decide that you like one thing or another. You have to listen to your gut. Who do you find attractive? Who do you enjoy spending time with? What do you like to fantasize about when you're masturbating? Who at school would you kiss if you could choose?

It's up to you to work out what you like. It is easiest if you can shut out all the external voices, so you can hear your own internal voice more easily.

Liking girls is just as valid as liking guys, liking both, or not wanting to have sex at all.

You don't have to decide

Some people find it easy to know what they like. They may have known all their life, just like Anders.

"I've never actually been in any doubt. At school I became interested in girls, and in high school I got together with my girlfriend and had sex for the first time. So I've never been conflicted and it would have been the same if I'd been gay," says Anders.

If you know what you like, you should stand your ground and not be swayed by others. You know best and you'll feel better if you follow your inner voice.

But you might find that you don't know what you like at first. Niklas was of two minds for a long time.

"It went in waves. Sometimes I thought that I liked guys, other times that I liked guys and girls. A big problem I had was that all the guys at school were so childish, so I didn't like any of them. Finally I worked out that I like people for who they are, not for their gender," says Niklas.

It's reported that four out of ten guys have had sexual experiences with other guys in their childhood and teens. The most common experiences are masturbating in front of each other, wanking each other off or sucking each other off. Some also experiment with anal sex. Most of the guys who do this are heterosexual, which shows that there is sometimes a difference between our sexual orientation and the sex we actually have.*

Not knowing what you like doesn't have to be a problem. You don't actually have to decide. It's perfectly fine to let love and horniness come to you from unexpected directions and let it surprise you.

Natural sexuality

I don't actually care about what's natural. Computers, video games, and glasses aren't natural, but I still use them.

But because some guys ask me what's natural, I'm going to talk about sexuality in nature.

Nature has plenty of examples that resemble the sexuality of humans. Many animals have sex for pleasure, not just to have babies. There are males who pair with females even when it's not mating season, so the female can't become pregnant. Many animals masturbate.

There are animals who have sex with others of the same gender. Same-sex intercourse occurs in animals such as wolves, hedgehogs, ducks, lions, hyenas, and dolphins. So far there have been studies of sexuality between two of the same gender in fifteen hundred species, but that figure is likely to increase, since research in this field is so new. Among some animals—for example, males in a pack of wolves— it's most common to have sex with someone of the same gender.

---

*Source: Shere Hite, *The Hite Report on Male Sexuality* (New York: Knopf, 1981), 45.

Glossary

HETEROSEXUAL	A guy who likes girls or a girl who likes guys
BISEXUAL	A person who likes both guys and girls
HOMOSEXUAL	A guy who likes guys or a girl who likes girls
STRAIGHT	Heterosexual
GAY	Guy who likes guys
LESBIAN	Girl who likes girls
ASEXUAL	Person who doesn't get aroused by or want to have sex with others
QUEER	An umbrella term for all non-hetero and non-cis identities

Love and sex between people of the same gender has been around forever, in every culture; it just hasn't been called homosexuality. Read the love story between the warrior David and Prince Jonathan in the Bible, for example.*

Animals sometimes choose to live with someone of the same gender. One interesting example is the black swans that live in Australia. Occasionally a male pairs up with a female, but once the eggs have

---

*Source: 1 Samuel 18–20.

hatched, the male chases the female away and another male moves into the nest. Cygnets that grow up with two dads have a better chance of survival than cygnets that grow up with a mom and a dad. For the black swans, there is therefore an evolutionary advantage to living as a same-sex couple.

In nature there are also animals that change gender, such as clownfish. And there are animals that never or almost never choose to mate.

Of course there's a big difference between sexuality in nature and sexuality in humans. In nature there are no labels. A wolf isn't going to say to another wolf "Ooh, you hetero, get lost!" And hedgehogs are never going to join in a Pride march. These animals don't see themselves as straight, gay, or bi.

The big similarity between sexuality in humans and in animals is that there is huge diversity.

Other people's expectations

When I was little, my parents sometimes asked me whether I thought a girl in school was cute or whether I was in love with a girl. At youth club, a boy might hit a girl and then one of the youth leaders would say it was because he liked her.

My parents never asked whether I thought a boy was cute. The youth leaders never claimed two boys liked each other because they'd had a fight. Not even every tenth time, which would at least have been statistically correct on their part.

Although quite a few of us youngsters were, according to the statistics, homosexual or bisexual, we were all treated as heterosexuals. And that's how we're treated throughout life.

> 88 percent of guys identify as heterosexual.*

Society expects everyone to be heterosexual, despite not everyone being straight and the fact that people do not choose to be straight or gay. This expectation crops up in every imaginable context, like when a relative asks whether you have a girlfriend but not whether you have a boyfriend.

This expectation is oppressive because it can make people who are homosexual or bisexual doubt themselves and feel bad. Throughout our lives, we're fed an image of who we should be, and when you discover you're different, you can feel like a failure, despite it being just as fine to like guys as it is to like girls.

Not necessarily obvious

Samuel is a sporty guy with a hoodie and cropped hair. I sit alone with him in the break room at his school and talk about love and designer clothes. Samuel thinks the way you look is important, and you can tell by his style. The clothes he's wearing have huge logos on them.

Samuel has had a few girlfriends, but he isn't sure whether he also likes guys. Maybe. But he doesn't understand gays.

"Why do they choose a style that makes it so obvious. Narrow eyebrows and so on? Why can't they look like everyone else?" says Samuel.

---

*Source: Sven-Axel Månsson, Ronny Tikkanen, Kristian Daneback, and Lotta Löfgren-Mårtenson, *Karlek och sexualitet pa internet* [*Youth and Sex on the Internet*] (Gothenburg and Malmo: Gothenburg University and Malmo University, 2003), 41.

One response to that question is, Why would people want to look like everyone else? Isn't it more fun to have your own style?

But another response is that Samuel can't know who is and isn't heterosexual. He guesses that guys who are campy are gay and guys who are more typically masculine are straight. But that may not be the case at all.

He is making his guesses based on certain expectations regarding heterosexuality. If we meet people who don't stand out in any way, we tend to assume that they are straight. But the statistics say otherwise. We actually meet gays and bisexuals all the time in school, at the gym, and at parties. Samuel meets many guys who are sporty like him and who are both homosexual and bisexual, but when he meets them Samuel assumes they're heterosexual.

"They probably also assume that I'm straight!" realizes Samuel.

Exercise: See diversity

Go to a place where there are lots of people, preferably people of different ages, with different amounts of wealth, and with different skin colors.

Count the people and accept that one in ten of the people you see is homosexual or bisexual to some degree. Whether the tenth person is an old man with a walking stick, a guy in a suit, or a girl with a veil, imagine that person as homosexual or bisexual.

This exercise opens up your eyes to the fact that people of different sexualities are all around you in everyday life.

The fear of difference

There are and have been societies where people are expected to have sex with others of the same gender. In such societies, no one raises an eyebrow if a guy likes another guy. In our society, everyone is expected to be heterosexual, so some people label homosexuality and bisexuality as "different."

Unfortunately it's in some people's nature to be afraid and suspicious of things that seem strange or different. That's why there are those who think it's wrong, strange, or disgusting that not everyone is heterosexual. These feelings are called homophobia, and you can be homophobic no matter what your own sexual orientation is.

> Our view of what is normal sex changes over time. In the 1940s many people thought it was perverse to suck on a woman's breast. This was something babies did, not men.*

Homophobia may be expressed through mean jokes, cruel comments, and bullying. Many homophobes fail to understand that they are surrounded by homosexuals and bisexuals all the time. Homophobes might, for example, tell a joke about homosexuals and think that no one's going to be upset, when in fact their best friend or brother might be gay or bisexual and will be hurt but will just keep quiet.

Because homophobia exists, many homosexuals and bisexuals feel

---

*Source: Alfred C. Kinsey et al., *Sexual Behavior in the Human Male* (Bloomington, IN: Indiana University Press, 1975), 371.

they can't be open. Take a look at your school. How many people there are openly gay or bisexual? The level of homophobia affects how open people can be.

Homophobia can be cured

Homophobia is a serious handicap, because you can't go around having a phobia about a large chunk of the population around you. Fortunately, homophobia can be cured.

Mahmoud works at a youth center, and he used to be homophobic.

"It was just something I was. I don't think I gave it much thought. I thought homosexuals were disgusting. I wasn't born here either. Where I come from its completely unacceptable even to have a gay friend," explains Mahmoud over a beer at a bar after the center has closed for the night.

> Guys who are uncertain about their sexuality tend to be the most homophobic. It is therefore no surprise that teenage guys become less homophobic over the years. Homophobia is basically something many people grow out of.*

The turning point came when Mahmoud and some of his friends went to Ibiza (an island off the cost of Spain that is a popular tourist destination). They'd been looking forward to the trip for a long time

*Source: Claes Herlitz, *Allmänheten och hiv/aids. Kunskaper, attityder och vanor* [*The Public and HIV/AIDS. Knowledge, Attitudes and Habits*] (Stockholm: Folkhälsoinstitutet, 1997).

and intended to party every day. At a bar, Mahmoud met a few gay people. At home he might never have talked to them, but now he was on holiday and in a good mood, so he went up and started chatting.

"They were great. We had so much fun together and we became friends. We partied and hung out a lot. There was nothing weird about them at all, they were just really funny," says Mahmoud.

And when he got back from Ibiza, his homophobia had been cured.

"Today I can sit chatting to someone who's gay and it's just normal, it makes no difference that he's homosexual. I like the way things are now," says Mahmoud as he orders another beer.

I've spoken to a psychology professor, who told me that homophobia is like other types of phobias. You have problems with something because you don't know much about it, and so you create scary images in your head. But if you get to know what you're afraid of, for example, by having a friend who is openly gay, that fear goes away.

BEING STRAIGHT

You may well decide that you only like girls. It's always good to know what you want, because then you can go and pursue it. But there's something you need to know. Homophobia isn't just there to oppress gay and bisexual people. Its main point is possibly to control heterosexual people.

Think about it. What is it that many straight guys want? It's for others not to think they're gay. Many people have said something mean about gay people at some time or other, even though they may not have really meant it. And you don't want people to say things like that about you.

And what do you have to do so that others won't think you're gay? Not stick out. In other words, play the male gender role.

Homophobia is treacherous because it makes straight people feel normal and maybe better than those who aren't straight. And it's nice to feel normal and better than others. But at the same time you become trapped and confined by homophobia, because as soon as you stop playing the male gender role, you're acting gay, and you don't want that because you thought being gay was bad.

So for your own sake, if you haven't already done so, try to rid yourself of any homophobia. It'll make you and the homosexual and bisexual people around you freer.

BEING GAY OR BI

If you realize that you're gay or bisexual, there are various ways you might react. You might have happy thoughts about all the great guys you could hook up with. Or you might be worried because all your life people have expected you just to like girls and now things haven't worked out like that. This can make you feel excluded or anxious about what your life is going to be like now that you're not living up to all these expectations.

If you are worried, I'd like to say a few reassuring words. Liking guys in the U.S. today is not like being gay in some other countries, or like it was in the past. If you want to, you can live your life much like everyone else: you can get married, have children and live together. The law says no one can stop you.

One upside to being gay or bi is that you're automatically going against some of society's expectations. And that makes it easier to choose paths other than the ones society has mapped out for you, if you so wish. You may not want children. You may want to spend your life traveling or completely rejecting the male gender role. This is all easier if you've already begun to walk a path other than the one staked out.

Facing homophobia

One thing that can make life really difficult is homophobia. You'll find homophobia all around you, whether you're out and proud or still in the closet. The homophobes may be other students, your family, teachers, priests, mullahs, and politicians on TV. They say horrible things that can make you feel terrible.

> "If I got to choose, I'd say it's better for children to grow up together with a woman and a man."
>
> A high-ranking Swedish politician blurts out his prejudice on TV. Why do some people think they have the right to criticize loving parents whom they've never met?*

It's good if you have a person you can talk to about these things. If you don't, try talking to a school guidance counselor or the people at your local youth clinic. Sometimes when you seek support, you'll encounter people who are homophobic and talk complete nonsense. In this case you should keep looking, because there is good support out there for people who are young and not heterosexual.

---

*Source: Anders Pihlblad, "Pihlblad Intervjuar: Kd-ledaren Göran Hägglund" ["Pihlblad Interviews: Christian Democrats Leader Goran Hagglund"] TV4, March 26, 2009, http://politikerbloggen.tv4.se/2009/03/26/pihlblad-intervjuar-kd-ledaren-goran-hagglund.

For someone living in an environment full of homophobia, this can sound like cold comfort, but everything tends to get easier with time. If your family or the place you live is unbearable, you can move away. You can ditch homophobic friends and replace them with people who like you for who you are.

It's probably at its worst for you right now, but thanks to smart moves on your part, things will get easier in a few years' time.

> Homophobia and the assumption of heterosexuality make it tougher to be gay or bisexual. This is why it is more common for gay and bisexual young people to suffer stress, anxiety, or suicidal thoughts compared with heterosexual young people.*

Perhaps the most important thing for you is not to let the homophobia take hold within you. It is all around you and it is hard to deal with, but it makes things even harder if you start to believe what others say and their thoughts become your own views. There are gay and bi people who convince themselves that not being straight is bad and that it's wrong not to keep to the male gender role. This makes it hard for them to like themselves and be happy.

Try being angry instead of sad. Be angry at being expected to be straight. Be angry at the existence of homophobia. Be angry at having to be sad. And join forces with other homosexuals, bisexuals, trans

---

*Source: National Alliance on Mental Illness, "How Do Mental Health Conditions Affect The LGBTQ Community?" accessed April 19, 2019, https://www.nami.org/Find-Support/LGBTQ.

people, and feminists to fight for a better society. Because things don't have to be the way they are today.

Getting to know others

It's common for gay and bisexual people to feel alone because they feel different or feel they're carrying a big secret. It's therefore good to get to know more people who are openly gay or bisexual, so you have something in common and can see yourself reflected in these people. This might also make it easier to find someone to fall in love with or have sex with if you want.

If there is a youth LGBTQ+ organization where you live, you should contact them. Everyone at GLSEN (Gay, Lesbian and Straight Education Network), for example, is very nice and they usually have loads of fun activities in the cities where they operate. The internet can also be a good way to get to know people, but as usual online, you have to be aware that sometimes people aren't who they say they are.

Try not to place too much emphasis on your sexual orientation. If you're bi and you meet another bi person, then yes you have one thing in common, but everything else could be completely different. You wouldn't expect two heterosexual people to get on just because they were both straight. If you try getting to know other gay and bisexual people with the attitude "Now I'm going to find others who think the same as I do," there's a risk that you'll be disappointed.

Just like everywhere else in society, homosexuals and bisexuals are subject to peer pressure. This pressure could relate to all sorts of things, but don't feel that you have to bow to it in order to be a "real" gay or bisexual. You actually don't have to have even kissed someone.

Meeting on gay dating apps

There are numerous apps for gay and bisexual guys. Search the word *gay* in your app store and you'll find them. These apps have an age minimum of eighteen because their main purpose is not for you to find friends and love but rather to hook up for sex. So, unfortunately, if you're younger, you'll have to wait until you're of legal age.

Hamza was thirteen when he downloaded the Grindr app. It was scary, and he deleted the app several times because he was afraid someone would discover that he had it. But the app was also exciting.

"I enjoyed looking at all the gay guys who were near me. When I walked around town, I kept hoping to see the guys, but I never did," says Hamza.

He had hoped to meet a boyfriend via the app, but instead an older man messaged him about sex and asked for naked pictures. He met up with a few men and had sex with them. Sometimes he felt good, but not always. One time a guy tried to force him into anal sex, so Hamza grabbed his clothes and fled from the apartment.

Step-by-step: How to come out

1. Try to get to know others via LBGTQ+ organizations like GLSEN, your school's GSA (Gay–Straight Alliance), or online. It's easy to come out if you know more people who are gay or bisexual.

2. Choose the person you come out to with care. Is it going to be someone who'll keep it secret or someone who'll pass it on? Many people choose to come out to friends and brothers or sisters before coming out to their parents.

3. Choose a place where you can talk undisturbed, preferably for a long time.

4. Explain that you're choosing to tell this person because you trust and value them.

5. If it goes well, you have a person who can support you and who you can talk to! If it goes badly, you have to remember that you are exactly the same person as you were before you came out. It's the other person who is doing the wrong thing, not you.

6. Since people are assumed to be heterosexual, it is unfortunately not enough to come out just once. Usually you have to come out again to new people you get to know, but it becomes easier with practice. When you're open, it increases the chances of people around you revealing that they are gay, bisexual, or transgender.

It is illegal to exchange sexual messages and pictures online with anyone under the age of consent. It may also be illegal to keep a naked picture of someone under the age of eighteen, because this may count as child pornography. Nice guys probably aren't lawbreakers. If you're under fifteen and someone over eighteen contacts you, they are therefore unlikely to be a nice guy. Hamza has also been given warnings like this, but they made him angry.

"Where else was I supposed to meet guys who were like me? I didn't know anyone who was openly gay and I hadn't told any of my family," says Hamza.

He has used various dating apps, including Tinder, but he doesn't use them anymore. He is now dating a guy and he's out to his family and friends. However, he thinks it's still hard to get to know gay guys, because many are so secretive.

"The best thing I ever did was to join an antiracism organization full of feminists. It was a great way to learn more about sexuality. The group Ungdom Mot Rasism (Youth Against Racism) was more important to me as a gay man than Grindr ever was," says Hamza.

To come out or not to come out

When Adam was in school, he felt it was impossible to come out about his sexuality. He had known his classmates for years, some of them since childhood, and Adam was afraid of being frozen out. But then he went to high school with completely different people.

"It was a special class with a focus on music, and even though I lived in a small town, many of the students moved there just to take this course. This meant many of them weren't living at home. You could be whoever you wanted to be in the class and there was a supportive atmosphere," says Adam.

The first time he told someone he liked guys, he was worried about what would happen.

"I texted a friend, 'I think I'm bi.' It turned out to be quite undramatic.

Then I told a few others, and at a party I made out with a guy. After that the rumor spread all through the school. A few friends dropped me at that point."

It took more than six months for Adam to come out to his parents.

"I was heading off to a festival, so I wrote a letter explaining everything. I left the letter where my parents would find it. I wrote that they shouldn't call me and that we could talk when I got home," explains Adam.

He thinks it's a good strategy to leave a letter behind if you're going away for a while. It gives everyone time to process the letter and no one does anything hasty.

"Mom called me anyway and said she loved me. When I came back from the festival we talked, cried, and argued."

It didn't all go well and he found a lot about coming out difficult. But according to Adam it was worth it.

"You get to live a freer life and feel better about yourself. I think you should do whatever it takes to be able to be yourself," says Adam.

You don't have to come out if you don't want to. You don't have to tell anyone. But if all goes well, coming out can be such a relief because, like Adam, you get to stop lying and hiding things.

7

SEX WITH GIRLS

WHAT TO DO WITH GIRLS

No matter who you want to have sex with, I think you should read about sleeping with girls and about sleeping with guys. Both chapters contain advice and exercises you might find useful, whoever you have sex with.

Guys often wonder what girls like. The fact that guys ask themselves this question is good, because it shows that they want the girl to have a good time.

And because it's such a common question among guys, there are also a number of books claiming that "this is what girls like." I don't want to take this approach because girls like different things.

When I interviewed girls about what kind of sex they enjoy, one girl told me she enjoyed receiving oral sex. Another girl hated it and didn't want any licking. It's clearly impossible to say that all girls like having sex in a particular way. The best thing is to listen to your sex partner's signals and follow their lead or ask them directly. That way you get to know what this particular girl likes. Sex is also not only about giving the other person what they want—you can also explore the other person's body for your own enjoyment. And you shouldn't do things you don't want to, just for the other person's sake.

Instead of trying to work out the "right" way of doing it, it's better to follow your desires. What do the two of you desire? Let your feelings guide you and do things that please and excite you.

But so as not to leave you completely high and dry, I'll be describing a few ways that you can have sex and giving you a few tips that I've gotten from my interviews with girls.

Things Not to Do!

- Try not to have sexual intercourse too quickly.
- Don't be selfish and decide everything yourself.
- If the girl is not wet, don't put saliva or anything else into the vagina and think that can take the place of her natural wetness. If she doesn't get wet, don't enter her vagina.
- Don't try and copy what they do in porn films.
- Don't do things too hard, at least not to start with.

Things to Do!

- Involve the whole of her body in the sex, for example, with caresses.
- Listen to what she wants.
- Care about both of you having a good time.
- Touch the outside of the pussy, don't just enter the vagina.
- Continue to be considerate even after the sex.

Caressing with your hands

There are many different ways of having sex, perhaps the simplest of which is to use your hands. You can get everywhere with your hands, so why not make the most of it. The sense of touch covers the whole body, so try touching more places than just the breasts and pussy. You can caress or massage.

If you or your sex partner don't like being naked, the hands are perfect, because you can have sex with them without taking off all your clothes.

When you use your hands to caress the pussy, you can try stroking the different parts to see what reaction you get. Try to learn how every part of the pussy feels against your fingertips and feel for any differences while you're stroking. Do you notice anything growing? Anything hardening?

If you notice wetness coming from the vagina, you can use this as lubrication for your fingers.

And just because you're caressing the pussy doesn't mean you have to stop stroking other places. You can switch between the pussy and other parts of the body. But don't stroke both the anus and the vagina with the same hand, as this could possibly give a girl a urinary tract infection.

Exercise: The name game

This exercise is a game you can play with a partner. The purpose of the exercise is to discover parts of the body you otherwise might forget to touch.

You should take turns "writing" the other person's name by kissing and stroking body parts that begin with the letter you want to write. For example, you can spell the name Sara by kissing and stroking: Shoulder, Ankle, Ring finger, Armpit.

Clearly some letters are harder than others. Be inventive, and if necessary you can cheat a bit with the spelling!

If you want to repeat the exercise, try doing it with middle names, family names, addresses, and so on.

Other ways to give hand sex

MASTURBATION

Instead of just caressing her, you can also try masturbating her by rubbing the clitoral hood backward and forward over the clitoral glans. You can do this with and without her lubrication on your fingers, but if you directly touch her clitoral glans without lubrication it can be an unpleasant sensation for her.

PRESSURE

You can try carefully applying pressure with your whole hand to the pubic mound just above the clitoral glans. You can also try gently pressing the labia to stimulate parts of the clitoris that lie inside the body. Ask where your pressure feels good.

FINGERING

If the vagina is wet, you can try carefully inserting a finger, a little at a time. Make sure you don't have long or sharp nails, and make sure your hands are clean, because if your hands are dirty it's possible to give her a urinary tract infection. There is a place where she might find it particularly pleasurable, and that's called the G-spot. The G-spot is an area a few inches inside the vagina, up toward the stomach, which feels rougher than the rest of the vagina. You can stroke this with a certain amount of pressure.

COPYCAT

If you really trust each other, you could ask her what she usually does when she masturbates. She might show you or guide your hand to pleasure herself. She knows what she likes best, so why not copy her movements?

With mouth and tongue

Having sex with the mouth can feel extremely close and intimate. It can therefore feel wonderful, but at the same time this closeness can feel excluding and therefore less pleasant. If you both want oral sex but are a bit unsure what to do, it's a good idea to take it slowly. Start with the thighs or stomach and approach the pussy at your own pace.

Don't see it as you having to perform. If you want to lick her, it's probably because you find it exciting yourself and because you like the intimacy. Work out what feels good to you.

> 93.9 percent of girls described the most recent time they received oral sex as a good experience.*

Don't waste this opportunity by doing the worst porn licking at a hundred licks a second. Take your time. Look around. Taste. Smell. Try licking in different ways: gently or with pressure, with a wide tongue or a narrow tongue. Check what reactions you get from the girl. In porn girls tend to be licked quickly and with the tip of the tongue, but when I've talked to girls about licking speed, that hasn't been the type of licking they've enjoyed most.

*Source: Elisabet Häggström-Nordin, Ulf Hanson, Tanja Tydén, "Associations between Pornography Consumption and Sexual Practices among Adolescents in Sweden," *International Journal of STD and AIDS* 16, no. 2 (February 2005): 102–7.

Tips: If you run out of ideas

- Don't just focus on one part of the pussy. Pleasure the girl over a larger area.
- You can suck as well as lick.
- Try inserting your tongue into the vagina.
- Use your hands as well. The fact that you're giving oral sex doesn't mean you have to stop sex with your hands.
- Try pulling up the clitoral hood and gently licking the glans.
- Sometimes it can be fun to give each other oral sex at the same time.

Frot

Rubbing your genitals against each other without the penis entering the vagina is called frot. You can do it in many different positions, but here are just two examples.

HER ON TOP

If you lie on your back with your legs together, the girl can sit on top of you, so her vaginal opening is resting against the shaft of your penis. Then you can both grind together. Both your and her genitals will be really aroused by this.

YOU ON TOP

If she lies on her back with her legs apart, you can lie on top of her with your own legs inside hers. It's easiest if she takes command and grabs hold of your dick. She can then rub your dick wherever it feels best for her.

SEXUAL INTERCOURSE

Not all girls can have sexual intercourse, partly because some girls don't find it enjoyable, and partly because some girls find it painful. You should never have sexual intercourse with a girl who finds it painful. The risk is that the nerves in the vagina will change so they cause more and more pain. Painful sexual intercourse can thus lead to a girl no longer being able to have vaginal sex.

> Six percent of girls between the ages of eighteen and twenty-four have experienced pain when trying to have sexual intercourse in the past year.*

Sexual intercourse is only a small part of sex with girls, so if the girl you're sleeping with can't or doesn't want to have intercourse, there are plenty of other things you can do.

But if you both want to and find it enjoyable, you can naturally go for it!

---

*Source: Bo Lewin, *Sex i Sverige : om sexuallivet i Sverige 1996 [Sex in Sweden: On Sex Life in Sweden in 1996]* (Stockholm: Folkhälsoinstitutet, 1998).

Different positions

Having sexual intercourse in different positions can create varied sensations for many people, because the penis enters at different angles and depths. It can therefore be cool to vary your sexual position.

But you shouldn't misunderstand this thing about sexual positions. I once read an article in a men's magazine claiming that the more positions you had sex in, the better you were in bed. They were suggesting that you should switch position ten times during sex in order for it to be good.

The guy who wrote the article and many other guys I've met think of sexual positions as a kind of performance, where you tick off as many as possible on a list. Instead of offering enjoyable variety, sexual positions become a theater number you have to rush through in your bedroom.

> About thirty percent of guys sometimes have sexual intercourse because it feels like it "has to be done." They would actually have preferred to skip the intercourse and have some other type of sex.*

I talk about sexual positions with a girl called Kristina.

"I call them 'circus performers.' They're the guys who throw you back and forth and do it every which way from different directions, as if they were acting in a porn film," says Kristina.

---

*Source: Shere Hite, *The Hite Report on Male Sexuality* (New York: Knopf, 1981), 1102.

Relax and stop making sex a competition to do as many positions as possible. Changing position can be fun, but it can also feel like an unnecessary interruption to the sex.

Here are a few examples of sexual positions.

COWGIRL

If you lie on your back with your legs together, the girl can sit on top of you and ride you. This is a position where the girl has control over the sex. You get a great view and can easily caress her breasts and stomach.

MISSIONARY

If the girl lies on her back and spreads her legs, you can lie on top of her and thrust. This position can be romantic, because it's easy to kiss or whisper things to each other. The girl can also easily caress your back and butt. To vary the position, the girl can lift one or both legs or raise her ass with a pillow. The same position can also be reversed, so the guy lies on his back with his legs together and the girl lies on top and thrusts.

DOGGY STYLE

The girl positions herself on all fours and you kneel behind her. In this position you can't see her face, so it's particularly important to listen to her signals to check she's enjoying it. It is easy for you to caress her back, buttocks, breasts, and stomach and massage her clitoris in this position. You can thrust quickly and hard without using up much energy.

SPOONING

Both of you lie on your side in the shape of a spoon, with you lying behind her. She parts her legs by lifting one of them and resting it on your leg. Now you can have sex from the rear. This position can feel extremely intimate and close, despite the fact that you're not looking into each other's faces. It's easy for you to caress her breasts, stomach, and clitoris.

Girls' Top 4 Sexual Positions*

1. Doggy style
2. Missionary
3. Cowgirl
4. Spooning

Guys' Top 4 Sexual Positions

1. Doggy style
2. Cowgirl
3. Missionary
4. Spooning

---

*Source: Online survey of 20,000 respondents on Swedish news site *aftonbladet.se*.

Take things slow to start with

In porn films, the guys often push in deep and quickly get thrusting right from the start. However, you should take things slow at the beginning of sexual intercourse if you are in control of the thrusting. Your dick is probably bigger than the fingers you've had inside her, and the vagina needs to adapt to the new size. Just insert a small part of your dick to start with.

Step-by-step: Having sexual intercourse

1. Make out and have other types of sex.
2. When she's properly wet, gently slide a finger into her vagina.
3. If it's her first time taking a dick, it can be a good idea for her to be on top so she can more easily control how deep the dick goes in.
4. Her legs should be apart. If they're together, there'll be no room for your dick.
5. The best way to insert your dick is to hold it in your hand; otherwise, it can be a bit tricky to get it "on target." You can also let her do it so it ends up at the right angle.
6. Only insert the top of the glans to begin with. Gradually thrust and slide deeper and deeper. It doesn't have to be the guy who takes charge of the thrusting.
7. The fact that you're having sexual intercourse doesn't mean you have to stop everything else. One of you can caress the clitoris during sex, for example.

8. If your dick slips and ends up near her anus, replace the condom or wash yourself before you continue with the sexual intercourse, so you avoid giving her a urinary tract infection.

9. You don't have to continue with sexual intercourse until you come. Sometimes, you may just want to have intercourse for a while and then move on to other types of sex. Maybe you could have intercourse later in the sex if you feel like it.

If the girl wants to take in more of your dick, you can do this gradually.

Sometimes girls might want things to be a bit rougher or are so horny and ready that the whole dick can be inserted quickly. But it's best to check with her first, instead of turning it into some kind of painful porn scene.

Premature ejaculation

Coming earlier than you want is a sensitive issue for many guys. After ejaculation, it's easy to lose your erection. Because the nerves in the dick need to rest, continuing with sex can also hurt. Many guys therefore want to be able to last a long time before they come.

Coming quickly is a sign of the pleasure you get from doing something you really enjoy. If you like continuing with sex after ejaculation, for example with your hands or mouth, the fact that you've come is irrelevant. You can simply carry on having sex without stimulating your dick.

When I began having sex, a friend gave me the tip that I should think of something utterly unsexy to last longer before coming. "Think of a rock!" he said. I did what he said. I thought about rocks while I had sex, my brain full of cold stone. And it worked in that it took me longer to come. But to be honest, having to think about rocks during sex is no fun. It gets in the way of the intimacy between you and the other person.

Exercise: Start/stop

This exercise is about you and the girl using your hands and mouth on each other at the same time.

When you feel you're about to come say "stop," so she ceases giving a hand job or oral sex. When you feel that your arousal has cooled a little and it's OK to continue, say "start," and the girl can begin giving sex again.

Try stopping the sex a few times. You might find you can have sex for longer than you thought without coming! You can also do this exercise on your own when you masturbate.

The problem of premature ejaculation can be solved by changing the way you have sex. Maybe it feels like you mainly come too early during sexual intercourse. The way the vagina surrounds the dick provides the guy with extreme stimulation, which makes him come very easily.

In this case, you can spend more time on making out, other types of sex, and games. This is likely to make the sex last longer. If you really want to have sexual intercourse, you could do it for a short time and then switch to other types of sex.

Focus on the moment, try to maintain the feeling of pleasure without rushing to the ejaculation stage. Over time it will get easier to control your ejaculation and not come until you want to.

When the girl doesn't orgasm

Usually, a guy thinks girls reach orgasm because of something he does with his dick, such as sexual intercourse. However the most common route to orgasm for girls is stimulation of the clitoris. If you think you come too quickly and the girl doesn't come at all, you could maybe review the sex. You might be putting too much focus on the vagina and too little on the clitoris.

Many guys bring the image they have of sex from TV with them into the bedroom. On film, girls often come very quickly and through sexual intercourse. A guy can therefore feel like a failure when he notices that the sex hasn't lived up to the image in his head.

With some guys, this feeling of failure leads to an obsession with the girl having an orgasm. There are girls who find it difficult to have an orgasm with another person and it's even more difficult if she feels under pressure. In the worst case, this pressure will lead to the girls faking their orgasms. Fake orgasms are bad for a relationship because they represent a breakdown in honest communication, and that makes it more difficult to improve the sex.

Instead of obsessing about orgasms, it's worth focusing on pleasure. Talk to her. What gives her pleasure? What would she like you to do to give her more pleasure? Build up a pressure-free atmosphere where she can relax and have a good time with you.

SEX IS FOR BOTH OF YOU

Erik remembers his first time. It was at his house with a girl who also hadn't had sex before. No one was home, but Erik locked his bedroom door just in case. After a while they ended up lying naked in bed.

"And she lay there on her back, not moving. So I lay on top of her and we had sex. But it was like having sex with a doll, really not cool," says Erik.

According to Erik, girls often lie down and expect him to do all the work.

"It's more fun with girls who take charge," Erik feels.

If you sleep with a girl and she just stays completely still, you should ask her what she wants, as she's not giving out any "yes" signals. The girl might be still because you're going too quickly, in which case you can rewind a bit and slow things down. You don't even need to have sex that time. You could make out and learn to relax together instead, so you can have sex some other time.

Unfortunately, one aspect of the male gender role is that guys are supposed to be sexual beasts. This sometimes means girls think that guys know exactly what to do and that she would come across as slutty if she took the initiative. Try to talk to each other, so the sex comes from both of you and you can find out what she wants. Sex is for the two of you, after all, not just one of you.

Equality in sex

As I've outlined before, we live in a society that is unfair to girls and where girls as a group have less power than guys as a group. It's therefore important that you make an effort to ensure that you and the girl you're in a relationship with are equal.

You've already learned how to do this. It's a case of listening to the signals, nobody having to do anything they don't want to, both of you getting to decide together, and you following the respect techniques. But it's also about sharing responsibility for your sexual health, for example, by grabbing some free condoms from the clinic and getting tested for sexually transmitted infections (STIs).

When you're on an equal footing, it's easier for both of you to relax and explore your sexuality without any shame.

Exercise: She decides everything

If you're sleeping with a girlfriend or regular sexual partner, you can play a game based on her deciding everything. If she says something, you have to do it. And if she doesn't say anything, you have to lie still and do nothing.

This gives the girl practice in making decisions and at the same time gives her a chance to work out what she really wants. The exercise also tells you what she likes and is up for.

The girl decides everything, but there is one exception. If she wants you to do something you're not comfortable with, say the safe word "red," and the two of you can move on to something else.

8 SEX WITH GUYS

EXPLORE

The fact that heterosexuals take up almost all the space on TV and in film is, for the most part, a bad thing. But there are advantages to being ever so slightly invisible. In sex between guys and girls there are many images to live up to. As a guy who sleeps with guys, you have more room to define your own sex and discover what you personally enjoy.

The sex guys mainly have with each other on film is anal sex. But when guys have sex, it usually doesn't involve penetration—simply because not everyone likes anal sex and those who do like it don't necessarily want it every time. Sex between guys can take whatever form you like, limited only by your imagination.

When you sleep with a guy, make sure you take the time to explore the whole of his body, not just his dick. There is so much more to a guy than what he has between his legs. Guys are sensitive to touch almost everywhere on the body, so run your hands or tongue over many different places.

You might think that because you're a guy you know exactly what other guys want. But guys aren't all the same. Let his signals guide you, and let him know when you enjoy what he's doing to you.

Not everyone is into the same thing

"Holding a dick feels different from guy to guy. I've noticed that they curve in different ways and vary in thickness. I never really thought about the shape of my own dick when I was jerking off; it just felt natural. But now I can see that it's curved, and I think about what other guys feel when they hold it," says Sumit.

Sumit says that he likes hand jobs.

"It's the easy option. Sometimes you're not up for anything more active, so you just jerk each other off."

He recalls discovering an interesting fact when he began having sex, which is that guys' dicks vary in sensitivity, and therefore guys masturbate slightly differently. Some jerk off gently, while others enjoy a harder action.

"Once I had a guy jerking me off and he was doing it so hard it hurt. When I told him, he admitted that he also didn't like the way I did it. He wanted me to grip it harder in my hand," says Sumit.

Tips for hand jobs!

- A hand job is about more than just masturbating. Feel the dick with your fingers. Caress it!
- Don't forget the scrotum. You can hold the scrotum and gently massage the balls backward and forward.
- Try gripping the base of the penis more firmly with just your thumb and index finger.
- Between the balls and the anus there is an area called the perineum. The erectile tissue that makes up the penis continues all the way down here. Pressing here can give a pleasurable sensation.
- Ask what he thinks about the speed and pressure when you jerk him off.
- Try giving a hand job with lube.

Oral sex

Oral sex is often called sucking off, but actually you don't need to suck particularly hard—it's not like sucking on a straw. It's enough just to suck gently or not to suck at all. When a dick enters the mouth, it's in a warm, moist environment that feels great. The most important thing is not to touch the dick, particularly the head, with your teeth.

97.7 percent of guys described the most recent time they received oral sex as a good experience.*

Having a dick in your mouth may not feel comfortable. It might feel too big or the precum might taste bad. In this case, it's worth bearing in mind that the head doesn't have to be in your mouth. You can lick wherever you feel the urge and suck on the shaft of the penis instead.

Exercise: Get it in deep

Being able to take a dick deep into your mouth can be cool, as it allows you to suck on as many of his sensitive nerve endings as possible. However, in the back of your throat you have a gag reflex, and nearly vomiting during sex is no fun.

Practice instead on a banana. You have masses of sensitive areas in your mouth, so try to trigger pleasant sensations on your lips and tongue using just the tip of the banana to start with.

When it feels good, you can try taking it farther and farther in and seeing if you can fool your gag reflex.

*Source: *Elisabet Häggström-Nordin, Ulf Hanson, Tanja Tydén, "Associations between Pornography Consumption and Sexual Practices among Adolescents in Sweden," International Journal of STD and AIDS 16,* no. 2 (February 2005): 102–107.

If he finds it difficult to control his ejaculation and you don't want cum in your mouth, you can use a condom.

Tips for giving a blow job!

- When you're going to put a dick in your mouth, make sure you open your mouth fully to keep your teeth away.
- Close your lips around the dick with a little pressure.
- You don't need to take it in very deeply if you don't want to or if you're afraid of gagging. Just suck on the head.
- You can jerk him off at the same time as you're giving him oral sex.
- You may not be able to get his whole dick in your mouth. But remember, you can reach everywhere with your tongue.
- Don't forget the scrotum. You can lick it or take a ball in your mouth and suck it.
- The area between the balls and the anus can be sensitive to licking.

Frot

When you lie dick to dick and rub them together, this is called frot. Frot is good because you can keep rubbing and still have your hands free for other things.

If you spread lube or saliva on the guy's dick, you can have frot with a better action. You can also hold both dicks and jerk them off at the same time.

Active and passive

Parts of the gay world use the words *active* and *passive* or *top* and *bottom*, which mean the same thing. The person being sucked off or doing the penetrating in anal sex is called active. The person doing the sucking or being penetrated is called passive. The words *active* and *passive* are thus used to describe who has their dick in whom.

But this is really the wrong way to use these words. When you suck someone off, you're very much the active party. Also, the so-called bottom can be active, for example, by riding the other guy's dick or by twisting his hips to affect the dick's angle of entry.

Some guys no doubt fit comfortably into one of these two categories, but often people will want different things at different times. One day you might fancy getting a blow job and the next you might really want to give one. So listen to your gut feeling and do what feels good in the moment, even if it's different from what usually feels good.

Not climaxing

"He was so hot and the sex was incredible. But I couldn't come," a friend tells me.

He is one of many who have spoken to me about the problem of not climaxing. Porn films often show close-ups of guys spraying away; they're used as some kind of proof that the sex was good and the guy enjoyed it. In bed guys are sometimes expected to do the same to show their appreciation.

But the difference is that porn films are edited. A porn actor might jerk off for several minutes while the rest of the film crew patiently waits for him to dump his load. Then they cut the film so it looks like the guy came exactly when he wanted to and when it was expected of him.

If you don't come, it's not a sign of failure or that you didn't enjoy yourself. Sex should never be a template that has to be completed the same way every time. You might have sex and climax sometimes, but it doesn't mean you always have to.

There are various possible reasons why a person can't reach a climax and ejaculate. One is that you may have been enjoying yourself but you've now had enough, for example, because you're tired or satisfied. In this case it's best to bring the sex to a close instead of forcing yourself to continue.

Another possible reason is that you've had good sex, but you have to take charge to reach a climax. Here you could, for example, jerk yourself off while your sex partner watches.

Yet another reason why you might find it difficult to climax is that you're putting too much pressure on yourself to perform the act of ejaculating, and that pressure is putting you off. In this situation, it's best to decide in advance that you aren't going to climax, so you can focus on the pleasure of the sex, rather than the pressure you're feeling.

9
MORE SEX

SEXTING

On the weekend Matteo works at a burger restaurant. Occasionally his mobile vibrates while he's at work. It's his girlfriend messaging him, usually something sexy. Matteo gets a thrill of excitement even before he reads what she's written.

"We talk about how we're going to have sex when we see each other. For example, she says she's going to strip me naked and lick my chest. Then I reply with what I'm going to do back," says Matteo.

The working day goes faster when they message each other. By the time they actually meet up, they're already so turned on that the sex feels even better.

Sending sexual texts and images to each other is called sexting. Matteo and his girlfriend do it to increase the excitement before they get together. But for many others sexting is a form of sex. They masturbate while they're sending the messages and they orgasm without having to meet up. Sexting allows them to have sex with people all over the world whom they would otherwise never have gotten to know.

The same age limit applies to sexting as to any other sex. A person over the age of fifteen must not make contact with someone under fifteen to suggest sex or ask for naked pictures. Doing so is called grooming. The law exists to protect young people from sexual assault.

Sending nude selfies

When Elliott was thirteen, he and a friend began sending pictures of their dicks to each other. They trained at the same gym, so they were used to seeing each other naked in the showers. By having pictures of his friend's dick on his phone, Elliott could compare their genitals in more detail. His friend began to develop pubic hair earlier than Elliott and their erections looked different.

"It was only then that I realized bodies vary. I used to think everyone was the same," he says.

For Elliott, photographing his dick soon became second nature. He snapped it in his room, in the bathroom, in school, and in his friends' bathrooms.

A few years later, Elliott entered high school. He became interested in a girl in a different class, so he asked his friends to talk to her. A few days later he got a text from the girl. "Hi, your friends said you were interested in me and they gave me your number. Show me what you have to offer."

Elliott thought long and hard about what she meant. It took him several days to work it out. Finally, he decided that she wanted to see his dick. So he pulled down his pants, took a selfie, and sent it to her.

The girl didn't reply. A photo of Elliott's dick was absolutely not what she wanted. Most girls don't want a photo of some random guy's dick, so it's not all that surprising. What she actually meant in her text was that Elliott should pluck up the courage to invite her on a proper date. She told Elliott's friends this. Afterward, Elliott did everything he could to avoid her at school.

> Only one in ten guys in senior high school have shown naked pictures of their body to others. It therefore seems that most guys who take naked selfies don't send them to anyone. Instead they use them to check themselves out.*

Time for a dick pic

Elliott waited until he was eighteen before he sent a dick pic to a girl again. This time he was sure she wanted it.

"Because we'd been sending scantily clad pictures to each other and she messaged that she wanted to see more," says Elliott.

It's actually not that difficult to know whether the other person wants a dick pic. First you send ordinary pictures to each other with sexy comments. If the other person sends a positive reply, you can move on to sending pictures with fewer clothes on; for example, a photo of you wrapped in a towel with the message "Just about to shower." If the other person sends back their own scantily clad

*Source: Linda Jonsson, "Online Sexual Behaviors among Swedish Youth," *European Child & Adolescent Psychiatry* 24, no.10 (October 2015): 1245–60.

pictures and sexy text, you can take the next step by asking something like "Do you want to see me without the towel?" If you get a yes, then it's time for a dick pic, but only then.

It's illegal to pull down your trousers and show your dick to anyone who doesn't want to see it. It doesn't matter whether this happens in the middle of town or via a text. A guy who sends unwanted dick pics is showing that he doesn't care about other people's boundaries. It's not nice.

Don't use your dick as a weapon to scare others. It can destroy your sex life when you later meet someone you love and want to have sex with. I've spoken to several guys who have had problems with sex because they've trained themselves to use their sexuality to degrade others by talking coarsely about girls, groping them, and sending unwanted naked selfies. Then when they meet someone they love, they find it difficult to change their view of what sex is.

Save your dick for those who want it—that way you'll enjoy the feeling that your body gives pleasure to others.

Four out of five girls between the ages of twelve and seventeen have received an unwanted dick pic, according to an online survey of 1,141 underage people. Some guys believe sex crimes are less serious if they're committed on a mobile phone, but that's wrong. Unwanted dick pics are illegal, and guys who send them can be reported to the police.*

*Source: *Dickpics*, directed by Ellinor Johansson, Josephine Jonäng, and Evelina Vennberg (Trollhättan: Folkuniversitets gymnasium, 2017), film.

Tips: How to take a good dick pic!

- Think about what can be seen in the background. Nothing ruins a sexy photo like attention-grabbing background items, like a toilet behind you or a hole in your sock revealing your big toe.
- Zoom out. Most people are interested in having a lover, not just a dick. So show more of your body. Have your dick resting on your stomach, show your legs as well or hold your dick in your hand, for example. That way you're showing that the dick is attached to a person.
- Use warm light, preferably sunlight or yellow light from an incandescent bulb. In particular, don't use the camera's flash or illuminate your dick with the light from a computer screen. That will make your skin pale blue, which looks scary. Is this a zombie sending dick pics?
- Don't show your face in the same picture as your genitals. That way you don't have to worry about being recognized if the other person's smartphone is stolen.
- The most important factor for the success of a dick pic is that the recipient really wants it.

RECORDING PORN

Some couples photograph or film their own porn to masturbate to when they're separated from each other. Others like to watch the porn together to get them horny before sex. There are many reasons to record your own porn, but there are even more reasons why people are not interested in making porn. Some people consider being naked far too private a thing to be photographed. Others find it hard work if it feels like you're shooting a film scene rather than being in the moment. There are also those who can't relax because they're thinking about the risk of the porn falling into the wrong hands.

Before you set up your camera, you therefore need to establish a few ground rules. First, do you both really want to record the sex, or does only one of you want to? Can either of you show the porn to other people? And what happens if one person wants the other person to delete the porn? Most relationships, whether between lovers or casual sex partners, end at some point. It's therefore good to decide in advance what you're going to do with the porn if you go your separate ways.

Some guys call it "revenge porn" when they publicly post porn involving a person who has dumped or rejected them. But people are perfectly entitled to end a relationship and to stop sleeping with someone. No one owns other people and so there is no reason for revenge when one person leaves another.

Filming or photographing someone naked secretly or against their will is illegal. It is also illegal to show or share naked images of a person who doesn't want that to happen. If you were under eighteen when you agreed to be photographed or filmed and the other person is now refusing to delete the images, you can report that person to the police for possession of child pornography. This will force the person to delete the porn.

There are ways to make porn other than with a camera. You can record the sound of you having sex to listen to afterward. (Note: Be ready for potential embarrassment!) Each of you can also write a sex novel featuring yourselves as the lead characters and then read them out to each other. Sometimes the sex novel might even become a reality. . . .

ANAL SEX

Anal sex is a type of sex that has many myths swirling around it. Whether or not you personally want to have anal sex, it's worth debunking these myths.

When they hear the words *anal sex*, many people automatically think of penetrative anal intercourse, where a dick or dildo is inserted into the anus. However, there is more to anal sex than just that.

Anal sex is not a new invention. There are vases from Ancient Greece depicting people doing it. Although awareness of anal sex has been spread via porn, it's clearly not a thing made up by porn actors.

Many question whether anal sex can bring any pleasure. And just like with everything else to do with sex, everyone has their own personal preferences. The body has the ability to take pleasure from anal sex, but this doesn't mean everyone enjoys it. The buttocks have nerves just like other parts of the body, so caressing a person's butt can bring pleasure and arousal. If a person inserts something into the anus, it can feel enjoyable because the sphincter muscles have sensitive nerve endings. If a guy is being stimulated in the anus, this also applies pressure to the prostate. If it's a girl, the action applies pressure to the female prostate glands and the clitoris.

Who you are doesn't determine whether you like receiving anal sex. Guys who like girls can be caressed and penetrated by girls using fingers or toys. Anal sex is by no means something that only guys who like guys can have. On the other hand, not all guys who like guys enjoy giving or receiving penetrative anal sex.

Sometimes when I talk to guys, they have an idea that the person being penetrated in anal sex is "split" somehow. But having anal sex is not dangerous. Nothing gets broken and it doesn't make it any more difficult to hold in your shit if you often insert fingers, dicks, or toys into your anus.

Using your hands and mouth

If you want to try anal sex, the best thing is to experiment a little and do what you think feels good and exciting. One approach may be to caress their butt with your hand. You can also stroke a finger backward and forward in their butt crack. The experience can be even more enjoyable if your finger is wet with lube or saliva.

> One in five eighteen-year-olds has tried anal
> sex at some point.*

*Source: Carl Goran Svedin et al., *Unga sex och Internet – i en föränderlig värld* [*Young Sex and the Internet – In a Changing World*] (Linköping: Linköping University Electronic Press, 2015), 17.

Another option is to insert a finger into the anus, but then you need to use plenty of lube and be very careful. Don't do it with long or sharp nails. The person receiving the fingering has to feel safe and relaxed, otherwise they will tense up and it will hurt.

You can also give pleasure with your mouth, for example, by biting gently on the butt cheeks or licking with your tongue.

When you part the buttocks and see the anus, you'll notice that it's darker than other skin. This is because there is more pigment here than elsewhere. The fact that it's darker has nothing to do with being unclean.

If you want to stimulate the inside of the anus but are afraid of getting dirty, you can roll a condom onto your fingers. But you won't usually get that dirty. When you insert a finger into the anus, the finger goes through a sphincter muscle and you end up in a passage of about four inches before the next sphincter muscle. There tends not to be any shit here unless the person needs to take a dump.

Anal intercourse

If you want to have anal intercourse, it's important to first have other forms of anal sex, so you get a chance to build up the sensitivity in the area. You should also stretch the sphincter muscle by inserting a finger in preparation for the penetrative sex. Use plenty of lube and place your fingertip against the anus, applying light pressure. The pressure makes it easier for the sphincter muscle to open. Once you've kept the pressure up for ten seconds, you can try carefully inserting your finger. Not the whole finger all at once, but slowly bit by bit. When you feel one finger is working well, you can insert another and then another. If it feels good for the person who is going to be penetrated, you can now begin the anal intercourse by inserting either a dick or a dildo.

Exercise: Understanding anal sex

Whether you want to give or receive anal sex, it's a good idea to try it out on your own first with a bit of anal masturbation. This will give you a better understanding of the pleasure that comes from inserting something into the anus. You'll learn how the sphincter muscle works and you'll discover how sensitive it is and how gently you have to progress with anal sex.

If you don't have a dildo, it's fine to masturbate with a carrot. Warm the carrot in water so it reaches a pleasant temperature, but don't let it go soft. Use a long carrot so you have a good grip on it when you masturbate. It's important to have a good grip so the carrot doesn't slip in and get stuck inside you.

Rub the whole area gently and use lube to stroke the anus. Roll on a condom and cover with plenty of lube. Press the carrot or the dildo against the sphincter muscle for a few seconds before you insert it. Try to relax and discover what feels good.

If you haven't done this before, ideally the person being penetrated should take control. The dick or dildo needs to enter at the correct angle and not go in too deep or too fast. If you are taking the dick or dildo, it's therefore best if you sit on top of the other person and let their dick or dildo enter you at the speed and to the depth that you want.

You'll come to a stop at around four inches in. There is another sphincter muscle here, and if the dick or dildo is to go any deeper, you'll have to do the same as you did with the first sphincter muscle.

The person taking the dick or dildo needs to relax as pressure is applied to the muscle for ten seconds before going in.

Anal sex should be a pleasurable experience. If it hurts, it's best to stop and try some other time. Forcing yourself through intercourse that hurts can create small tears in the rectum.

If you lose your erection while being penetrated, it may be simply because the blood is flowing to the sphincter muscle, which makes it difficult to continue keeping your hard-on. So you can be enjoying yourself and feeling aroused but still lose your erection during anal sex.

Making it work

Many people I talk to feel that anal sex went badly the first time they tried it. Magnus recalls how he had given anal sex and looked forward to receiving it.

"The sex was great until he stuck it in. I wasn't prepared for it to feel so big and rock hard! He stuck it in a few times and I said okay, that's enough," says Magnus.

Half of girls in their last year of high school who have had anal sex thought it was a bad or very bad experience. Anal sex requires knowledge and practice to work. And as with every other kind of sex, both people must really want it.*

*Source: Elisabet Häggström-Nordin, Ulf Hanson, Tanja Tydén, "Associations between Pornography Consumption and Sexual Practices among Adolescents in Sweden," International Journal of STD and AIDS 16, no. 2 (February 2005): 102–107.

It was a long a time before Magnus tried again.

"It's better now, but it's still not perfect. I really want to make it work, because it's really hot for the guy doing the giving, and that's how I want to have sex," says Magnus.

If you've longed to receive anal sex but have not managed to enjoy it, you can be left feeling rather deflated. But anal sex is a more complicated form of sex that can require practice.

When you have sex, don't focus so much on the penetration. Have other types of sex, and if you then really feel up for anal sex, you can try it. It's best if you take charge to begin with. And remember that you don't have to have the anal sex for long if it hurts. Carry on for as long as it feels good, and when you want to do something else, you can simply switch.

TALK ABOUT SEX

You must communicate about sex. It's how you find out whether the other person is giving their consent, but communication is also how you make sure both of you have a good time. Instead of looking for a sex technique that "everyone enjoys," you can follow your own horniness and your sex partner's signals and find something that works for the two of you.

If you frequently sleep with the same person and you trust each other, you can try talking about your sex. One good way of starting the conversation after sex is to say something you enjoyed and ask whether there was anything your sex partner particularly liked.

You can also ask whether your sex partner wants you to do anything differently. If, for example, your sex partner asks you to caress them more gently next time you have sex, you can ask, "Is this what you meant, or even gentler?"

By talking about sex, you can develop your sexual relationship and make it perfect for you two.

When you talk about sex, don't use phrases like "That was bad." You're not trying to knock each other's confidence, so try to find a way of talking that keeps you both feeling positive.

Getting stuck in a rut

Sometimes you can find yourself repeating the same kind of sex time after time. It can happen when you've been going out with or sleeping with someone for a while. But it can also be that you do the same kind of thing with every one-night stand, even though each one is a different person.

If things are getting boringly repetitive, you can always switch things up a little. If you have one-night stands, it's up to you to have sex in different ways. But if you have a partner or friend with benefits, you can talk about it. What do you always do? Then you can agree to ditch that type of sex for the next few times. If you have sexual intercourse all the time, for example, you could decide that you're not going to do that the next three times you have sex. You then automatically have to find other ways of having sex.

You can also do the exercise below, where you write lists. There are probably all sorts of things you both enjoy and haven't done for a while because you've simply forgotten about them.

If you're open with each other, you can continue to be loved up and have great sex with each other after many years together!

Exercise: Explore your fantasies

This exercise is for those of you who are in a long-term sexual relationship and would like to enact your fantasies. You and your sex partner can each write a list of your personal fantasies. These may be things you want to happen or places you want to have sex in.

Then you can compare lists. Is there anything that appears on both lists? Are there things on the other person's list that you would like to add to yours? Are there things you would dare to do with each other, or is it best if they continue to be a fantasy?

It's important to be open to the idea that you may like different things. You may want to try something your sex partner really doesn't want to do. This doesn't mean there's anything wrong with your fantasies or that wanting to do a certain thing is bad. You're simply two different people and you don't need to do anything except what you both enjoy.

FEELING GOOD

10

EMOTIONS

Sex can make you feel good or bad. If you ever find that sex or your sexuality is making you feel bad, you should sit down and think about what feels wrong. Try having sex in other ways or thinking differently about your sexuality. Find a path that leads you to feel good.

One of the most common sources of bad feelings about sex is that you pressure yourself to be good in bed. You want to show that you know all about sex and that you can pleasure the other person. It's not a bad thing to care so much about your sex partners. You need to care in order for both of you to enjoy it. But it goes too far if you have performance anxiety or begin to compare yourself with how good others are in bed.

There are many reasons why you might get performance anxiety. One might be that you go into sex believing that you have to live up to a set picture of what sex should be like. When the sex doesn't live up to that picture, it makes you unhappy. If this happens to you, try to be present in the sex instead of thinking about list items that have to be ticked off. Talk to your sex partner, as maybe you're trying to live up to an ideal that your sex partner couldn't care less about.

Another cause of performance anxiety can be low self-esteem. If generally you find it difficult to believe you're good enough, it can lead you to think you're bad in bed. If you trust your sex partner, you can talk about this. It may make you feel better to know that your sex partner is less critical about you than you are about yourself. In the long run, the solution is to tackle your self-esteem issues, maybe with support from an adult.

Shame and guilt

There's a set picture of what sex should look like, and it's extremely limited compared with how many different types of sex and sexuality there are out there. At some point, most people will compare themselves with this picture and think, *I'd like to try doing it a different way, does that make me weird?* The set picture can easily lead you to feel different. And because we don't usually talk about these things, it might well seem like you're the only one who feels this way.

If you ever feel ashamed about the sex you have or want to have, it's important to understand that although the feeling of shame is inside you, the shame actually comes from the world around you. The picture of how sex should be and other people's opinions about what is right and wrong have been fed to you since you were little. Your sexuality may be shameful by other people's standards. But you should ignore their standards and decide for yourself what is right and wrong. As long as there isn't an illegal difference in age, you aren't harming anyone, and everyone involved is happy, it's just one more good way of having sex.

There are some people who spend much of their life feeling ashamed. They may have sex and enjoy it at the time, but as soon as the sex is over, the shame comes creeping in and they try to stop thinking about it. Until the next time they have sex. The shame is like a wheel that just keeps on turning because you don't dare tackle the problem. Shame can prevent you from accepting that it feels good, so you might think you need to drink to have sex or turn the sex into something destructive.

If you feel ashamed, you should take a stand and admit to yourself that you like what you like. You have to be courageous about standing up for the person you are. That way you can fight the shame and enjoy sex without having to feel bad about it afterward. Sometimes it can make things easier to talk to a therapist, for example.

Going against your gut

As I've written before, guys don't always want to have sex. You have a gut feeling that sometimes says yes and at other times says no. It can happen that guys go along with sex despite the gut saying no.

There are many reasons why guys might pursue sex, despite not really feeling it. It could be that you want to have sex but you can't find someone you like to do it with, so you have sex with a person you don't really like, just to try it out. You might do it to look macho in front of your friends. You might be in a relationship and afraid that it might come across as not being in love anymore. Maybe it felt good to begin with and you feel guilty about stopping what you started, despite the good feeling having gone. If you have low self-esteem or feel bad, you may pursue sex to punish yourself by doing something you don't actually want to do or because you feel you don't deserve any better.

Whatever your reason for having sex despite not wanting it, you're not being good to yourself. It's important to listen to your feelings, because if you don't, there's a risk you'll end up being unhappy or feeling bad.

Only you can know exactly what your gut says and make sure you only go along with sex if you really want it. Because you're a guy, and the male gender role says that guys always want sex, only you can stop yourself from having sex you don't want.

If you find it difficult to set limits or to know where your limits are, it's worth talking to a professional adult, such as a doctor or therapist.

Being forced into sex

Guys are sometimes subjected to sex against their will. This is not something that gets talked about very often. Sex with force doesn't have to be particularly violent. It's common that people forced into having sex are so surprised by what's happening that they become silent and motionless, unable to put up any resistance or say no. Force can also occur in a situation where you can't say no, such as when you're really drunk, under the influence of drugs, or sleeping. And the perpetrator can be anyone, regardless of gender identity, sexual orientation, age, or their relationship to you.

You can get an erection even when you aren't horny, for example just because someone is touching your penis. This means you can get an erection even when you're being subjected to something against your will. It can also feel nice to some extent when someone does things to your body that you don't want. Guys can sometimes find it hard to understand that they've been subjected to force. After all, they had an erection and maybe enjoyed it a little even though they would rather it hadn't happened.

It's most common for girls to be subjected to sexual assault, but it also happens to guys. One in eight guys in the second year of high school have had their body touched when they didn't want it. One in fourteen guys have been subjected to intercourse against their will.*

I talk to a guy I know called Lars. He once went home with someone he wanted to have sex with. But when they got to the apartment, the atmosphere turned violent and Lars was raped. Afterward, he thought people wouldn't understand how a guy could be raped.

"It doesn't fit with the male image. In the media, men are dangerous and can commit rape. But you don't really hear about men being raped. This makes you think what happened was your own fault, but it's never your fault," says Lars.

Lars didn't report the rape to the police. Guys rarely report assault, so it's also difficult to know how many men it happens to.

---

*Source: Cecilia Åslund et al., "Shaming Experiences and the Association between Adolescent Depression and Psychosocial Risk Factors," *European Child & Adolescent Psychiatry* 16, no. 5 (August 2007): 298–304.

If you've been forced into sex, whether it's now or as a child and whether it felt horrible or not, it's good to talk to someone about what happened. There are some burdens you shouldn't bear on your own.

Someone to talk to

Sometimes it's good to talk instead of keeping things inside. You can speak to a friend, someone in your family, an adult in your life, or a professional on a support line you've called. You can also turn to a professional you meet in person at school or at a doctor's or therapist's office. Not everyone is an equally good listener. If you've tried talking to someone and it hasn't worked, it's important to keep looking until you find someone who can provide support.

I talk to Simon, who works as a therapist at a youth clinic and deals with many young men. He explains that the guys often don't know that they feel bad or don't understand why.

"They usually come to me because they have a physical problem or believe they've caught a sexually transmitted disease. But when I start asking them how they are, they say things are difficult at home or they're worried about the future and other things," says Simon.

According to Simon, you might not notice that you're not feeling great, because the feeling has developed over a long period of time. It's therefore good to talk to someone, as it provides an opportunity to put what's happening into words. Sometimes emotions can take a form different from crying—you might sleep with lots of people or drink or get angry, all the time not realizing that this may be rooted in the fact that you're not feeling good.

"Does not feeling good affect your sex life?" I ask.

"Yes. Many guys have problems in bed that they want to talk about, and they don't see that the problem may be linked to other feelings. If you enjoy life less because of something that's happened, clearly that's going to affect your sexuality. Sometimes it can lead to a vicious circle. You feel bad and then you get even more down when you can't make sex work the way you want. At that point, it's important to stop and get help with sorting through all your thoughts and emotions by talking to an adult.

SAFER SEX

I think sex is cool and something that makes me feel good. Sex can also make a relationship I have with another person even better and closer. I have a positive relationship with sex and I want that to continue.

However, sex can easily be a source of anxiety instead. If, for example, you wake up one morning next to someone and think, *Shit, what do I do now? Do I have a sexually transmitted disease? Do I have a baby on the way?*, then sex quickly goes from being fun to being a real problem. Because I don't want sex to feel like a problem, I have safer sex.

Sex can never be 100 percent risk-free. Condoms can break and a plane could drop out of the sky when you're having sex. But there are a few simple ways to make sex much safer.

Make a decision

Only you get to decide whether you have safer sex. If you want to be safe, you must make sure it happens and you must do it for your own sake, not because the health department says so or because you read it in a book.

The best way is, in a sober state, to sit down and think about whether you think it's worth the effort to have safer sex. Starting to think about safer sex when your trousers are down is far too late, as by then you're not thinking clearly. The decision has to be made earlier than that.

There are many reasons for choosing safer sex. One key reason is that the sex is more enjoyable if you can focus on it completely, without having that nagging doubt in the back of your mind that you're making a mistake. Afterward, you also avoid the potential worry or consequences.

Eight out of ten fifteen-year-olds used a condom when they last had sex. The younger we are, the more careful we are about having safer sex.*

You can't tell by looking at a person whether they are free from sexually transmitted infections (STIs), even if you meet the person at church and they look angelic. By sleeping with someone without protection, you're also sleeping with all the other people they had unprotected sex with previously, and you know nothing about them.

How STIs work

There are entrances and exits in the body that are called mucous membranes. When two people's mucous membranes touch each other, an STI can be transmitted from one person to the other. STIs

---

*Source: Karin Edgardh,"Adolescent Sexual Health in Sweden," *Sexually Transmitted Infections* 78, no.5 (October 2002): 353.

can also be transmitted if semen or blood from one person comes into contact with the mucous membrane of the other person.

The mucous membranes you should think about when having sex are the dick, pussy, anus, mouth, and eyes. If you protect your mucous membranes, you're protecting yourself against most sexually transmitted infections, including HIV.

Sometimes I talk to guys who think you can get HIV if you have a little old cut and get HIV-positive blood on it, if you get pricked by a drug user's needle, or if you're stung by a mosquito that has just sucked blood from someone with HIV. There are also those who believe you can get chlamydia from a toilet seat. Not one of those notions is true. Sexually transmitted infections can't survive outside the body, so you need not worry about STIs other than when you're having sex.

Ways to make sex safer

If you want to have safer sex, I suggest two possible safety levels.

I call the one level "safer," and that's based on you trying to avoid the *most* common ways that STIs are transmitted.

I call the second level "even safer," and that's based on you also trying to avoid *less* common ways to catch an STI.

This is what you can do to make sex safer and even safer.

HAND JOBS

Safer: Hand jobs are safer sex and cannot transmit HIV.

Even safer: When you're giving someone a hand job, try to avoid rubbing your eyes or touching your own genitals with the same hand.

ORAL SEX WITH A GIRL

Safer: Avoid getting menstrual blood in your mouth or eyes, as HIV can be transmitted through blood. If you do want to lick a girl during her period, you can cut up a condom so you get a rectangle, place it against the pussy, and lick. You can also use plastic wrap.

Even safer: Use a cut-up condom, a dental dam, or plastic wrap even when she isn't on her period.

Some people are allergic to latex, which is what most condoms are made from. To avoid the problem, you can instead use plastic condoms, which are also better at conducting heat. They're available from your school nurse or local pharmacy.

ORAL SEX WITH A GUY

Safer: Don't get semen in your mouth or eyes, as HIV can be transmitted via semen.

Even safer: Use a condom when giving a blow job or avoid putting the glans in your mouth if you're not using a condom, as there is a small risk of getting an STI from the precum or from contact with the urethra.

FROT

Safer: Frot (sexual rubbing) is safer sex and cannot transmit HIV. Avoid contact with semen during frot.

Even safer: Use a condom during frot.

VAGINAL INTERCOURSE

Safer: Using a condom protects you not only against sexually transmitted infections such as HIV and chlamydia but also against unwanted pregnancies. The pill and other contraceptives protect against pregnancy but not against STIs.

ANAL SEX

Safer: Use a condom and plenty of lube. If you don't have any lube, don't replace it with skin lotion, as that can make the condom break. If you really want anal sex, in an emergency lots of saliva can work, but saliva dries out quickly, so always try to keep condoms and lube with you if you enjoy anal sex.

HIV and chlamydia

There are many sexually transmitted infections, but I'm going to tell you about two of them that you should be particularly aware of.

HIV is incurable and attacks the immune system. Over a few years, the immune system becomes so weak that you reach the stage known as AIDS. At this point you contract infections easily and risk dying from them as a result of the body's inability to fight them off.

Antiretroviral therapy prevents HIV from developing into AIDS, so HIV is no longer a death sentence, at least if you live in a rich country. People on antiretroviral therapy have to regularly measure how much of the virus they have in the body. With successful treatment, the levels of the virus may go down so far that the person can no longer transmit HIV to another person through sex. This is known as untransmittable HIV.

Chlamydia is not as dangerous as HIV, but it's much more common. It often has no symptoms. You can carry the infection around for many years without knowing it, which could lead you to become infertile. Chlamydia is the most common reason young people in Sweden are unable to have children. It's also easier to get HIV if you have chlamydia. But if you know you have chlamydia, it's easy to cure.

Generally speaking, with the exception of HIV, other infections can be cured or are not very harmful. Since STIs are largely transmitted in the same way, having safer sex protects you against all of them at the same time.

There are, however, some infections that can be transmitted even though you have protected sex. Pubic lice (crabs) are one example. They itch but are otherwise harmless. You can get rid of pubic lice with special creams and shampoos. Another infection that safer sex won't stop is oral herpes, which is transmitted by kissing. Oral herpes is harmless. Mouth ulcers are a symptom, but most people don't get ulcers when they have oral herpes. If you do get one, the pharmacy has medication to deal with it.

Since you can't do much to protect yourself against these infections, I don't see any point in worrying about them. Instead, you should focus on the infections that you can avoid through safer sex.

Practice makes perfect

Condoms provide good protection, whether you want to avoid HIV or chlamydia or pregnancy. Today, condoms have a bit of a nerdy rep, since if you use them, you're seen as a "good boy." But don't forget that condoms have been around for less than a hundred years. Before then, people often contracted syphilis or other infectious diseases if they wanted to sleep around. Guys who liked girls became fathers practically as soon as they began having sex. Condoms now mean that everyone who wants to have sex can do so without most of the unwanted consequences. There are also people who are allergic to semen, and they need condoms to have any sex at all.

There is also a kind of medication that helps keep you from getting HIV. PrEP (pre-exposure prophylaxis) is a pill you take every day that, if taken consistently, can reduce your chance of contracting HIV by 90 percent if you are exposed to the virus.* If you're at high risk of exposure, it's a good idea to take it.

I speak to a guy named Thomas about condoms, and he thinks they're easy to use.

"Putting one on during sex has worked well. That might be because I've practiced quite a lot on my own, putting a condom on and rubbing myself against the sheets. So when I started having sex, I knew the practicalities," says Thomas.

He doesn't have a problem with rolling a condom on when he's sleeping with a one-night stand. It feels about as good as without a condom, particularly now that he's begun using an extra-thin kind.

However, he finds it more difficult to use a condom with someone he's interested in, because then Thomas really wants to come across well.

---

*Source: Centers for Disease Control, www.cdc.gov/hiv/basics/prep.html.

"You don't want to seem boring. You want to be passionate, and taking out a condom doesn't fit with that picture," says Thomas.

It's common to worry about what other people think when you take out a condom. But studies have shown that both girls and guys think it's good when the person they're going to sleep with takes the initiative to use a condom.

However, Thomas thinks the most difficult thing about using a condom is the interruption when he has to put one on.

"We're making out and I have an erection, and then I have to put on a condom. I sometimes start thinking, *Is it going to be hard enough?* Then the moment's gone and I lose my erection," says Thomas.

Thomas says the problem is actually in his head, not with the condom. And he has two ideas about how to try and resolve this issue.

"I've tried asking the other person to roll a condom onto me. If it's done well, it can be woven into the sex and I think that's one solution to the problem. But my other idea is to put a condom on earlier and make out with it on. That way there's no interruption when I'm going in," says Thomas.

I think you should follow Thomas's example. Practice putting on a condom before you have sex, so it becomes second nature. Try different condoms and find the one that suits you and your partner best. And try to make putting on the condom part of the sex—preferably something you do together. If the person you're sleeping with isn't used to putting on condoms, you can show them what you want them to do.

If you're going to have sex and you find you don't have a condom with you, get a hand job or engage in frot or oral sex instead of penetrative sex to avoid worrying afterward.

Step-by-step: Putting on a condom

- The condom pack has a little triangular nick in the middle. Make a small tear here and then break open the pack.
- Place your thumbs inside the condom and roll it a little with your index fingers. That will tell you whether the condom is turned the right way or whether it is inside out. Make sure it's the right way before you place the condom over the glans.
- If you have a foreskin, pull it back. The foreskin makes it easier for the condom to move. If you're circumcised and find condoms often break, try putting a little lube or saliva on the glans to make the condom more mobile, then it won't wear through as easily.
- While pinching the small part sticking up at the tip of the condom, use your thumb and index finger to press out all the air when you place the condom on the glans. Guys sometimes report that their condoms break, and this can often happen because there is air between the condom and the penis. Also be careful that nails, rings, or teeth don't break the condom.
- Roll out the whole condom. Condoms are a few inches longer than penises, so when you've rolled it all the way down to the root of the penis, form a circular grip with your thumb and index finger and pull the condom a little

way up the penis. Then roll the condom down the extra
bit. The condom will end up being slightly wrinkled.

- If you come while inside someone, hold the condom at the
penis root when you pull out. The hardness of your erection
can reduce quickly after ejaculation, and there's a risk that
the condom could come off in the other person if you pull
out without holding on to it.

Get tested for infections

Having safer sex isn't just about what you do in bed but also about
having a routine for getting tested for sexually transmitted diseases.
Get yourself tested at least once a year. If, despite your safety mea-
sures, you do catch an STI, it's good to find out early and get medical
attention.

Sometimes, you may end up having unsafe sex for whatever reason. Then you should contact your local youth clinic and book a test.
You often won't have any symptoms when you've got an STI, so you
can't be sure that you're healthy unless you get tested.

I remember the first time I got tested. First, I went and sat in the
waiting room, where the atmosphere was a little tense. I buried my
head in a newspaper and tried not to be noticed by the others there.
Soon my turn came around.

I had to pee in a test tube. Peeing was a relief, as I had been told not
to pee for a few hours before my appointment. Then I had to take another test that involved sticking a cotton swab into my urethra. The
nurse was going to do it for me, but I was scared that it might hurt so I

asked to do it myself. She told me what to do and I took the test. Sticking the cotton swab in stung a little but it wasn't exactly traumatic.

The nurse also took two different swabs from my throat. It's important to be clear about what kind of sex you've had. Sexually transmitted infections such as chlamydia and gonorrhea have to be tested for in the place where the STI would have been caught, so in the penis, anus, or throat.

The final test was a blood test to check whether I had HIV.

One week later, I returned to the clinic to find out whether I had any sexually transmitted diseases. It felt good to find out that I was fully healthy.

PREGNANCY

Because sex generally involves two people, you have to share responsibility for the sex being safe. You can't put the responsibility on the girl and expect her to take out a condom or take the pill. Accepting your share of the responsibility for preventing pregnancy is a way of taking responsibility for both of you feeling good during and after intercourse.

I have heard guys say that if you have sex but don't come inside the girl, she can't get pregnant. But if it was that simple, we wouldn't have needed to invent condoms and contraceptive pills, would we? One in five of those who try the withdrawal method end up pregnant within a year. This is mainly because guys aren't as good at controlling their ejaculations as they think they are. If you want to have sex without a condom, agree instead that you both will get tested for STIs, and then the female can start using an IUD or some other contraceptive.

Some people also talk about "safe periods" when girls can't get pregnant. Tracking these cycles is sometimes called the rhythm method of birth control. But these periods are actually not easy to pin down. Girls' menstrual cycles are also not always regular, and young girls in particular can have rather irregular cycles. In addition, sperm can survive inside a girl for several days, with fertilization often occurring a day or more after the sex. Of those who try to pinpoint these safe periods, a quarter become pregnant within a year. Safe periods are clearly a very unsafe method.

If, in the heat of the moment, you've had unprotected sex and the girl wants to avoid pregnancy, she needs to take the emergency contraceptive pill (morning-after pill) or insert an IUD (coil) as soon as possible. A girl can take emergency contraceptive pills up to five days after sex, but the earlier she does, the lower the risk of pregnancy. Emergency contraception can only stop a pregnancy from happening in the first place. If the pregnancy has already begun, they have no effect.

Approximate effectiveness of emergency contraceptive pills:*

95 percent if taken within twenty-four hours of sex
85 percent if taken within two days of sex
58 percent within three days

*Source: Charlotte Ellertson et al., "Emergency Contraception: A Review of the Programmatic and Social Science Literature Contraception," *Contraception* 61, no. 3 (March 2000): 145–86.

Emergency contraceptive pills are no replacement for regular contraception. If you take them more than once a month, their effectiveness can drop.

A good way to share the responsibility if you've had unprotected sex is to both go to the pharmacy to buy the pill, then split the cost.

Abortion

If a girl gets pregnant, she and the guy have a shared responsibility, as they were both involved in getting her pregnant. But because the pregnancy takes place in the girl's body, she gets to decide whether she wants to continue with it or have an abortion. Both pregnancies and abortions can be difficult things to go through, so it has to be up to the girl to decide what she wants to do. Many guys might find it tough to leave such a life-changing issue in another person's hands. That's why safer sex is so important as a way of having power over your own life.

If the girl decides to have an abortion, you should share responsibility for it. If you're going through with an abortion, ask the girl what support she needs. She might want you to go with her when she has the procedure and to be there when she's recovering afterward. You can be supportive by being there for her and paying attention to her thoughts and feelings.

If you're together, the abortion doesn't have to spell the end of your relationship. I know many couples who have been through an abortion and stayed together. The way you react to the abortion can be critical in determining what happens afterward.

Contraception

If you want to have unprotected vaginal sex but without the risk of having children, you need contraception. There are all sorts of contraceptives, which suit different kinds of people. To get the best advice, book an appointment with your doctor to talk about your situation or talk to your school nurse or guidance counselor. Sometimes a girl might need to try several different contraceptives before she finds the one that works best for her.

The alternatives to a condom are not problem-free. They can give the girl headaches, a reduced sex drive, acne, and even dangerous blood clots. You therefore can't assume that a girl will want to use other contraception instead of condoms.

Responsibility

To start with, thinking about condoms and getting tested can seem like hard work. In the moment, you may be too horny or too drunk for things to go the way you intended.

But in the long term it's worth working to achieve the kind of sex that allows you to relax afterward and not worry. It's a way to look after yourself, and taking responsibility for your sex life will make you feel good. By shouldering this responsibility, you're taking a step toward adulthood.

RESOURCES

AHA FOUNDATION

www.theahafoundation.org

The Ayaan Hirsi Ali Foundation works to prevent honor violence, forced marriages, and female genital mutilation. They maintain a list of organizations in each state that help victims of honor-based oppression on their website. They operate an emergency text line for anyone suffering from honor-based oppression that connects them with a counselor (text FREE to 741-741).

A CALL TO MEN

http://www.acalltomen.org

A Call to Men is an organization that talks about the male gender role and works to combat male violence.

GLSEN

www.glsen.org

If you're a young gay, bi, trans, or queer person, you can meet others like you through GLSEN, which has chapters across the country. In addition to organizing activities in schools, they fight for a society in which different sexualities and gender identities are treated equally.

PLANNED PARENTHOOD

www.plannedparenthood.org

Planned Parenthood is one of the largest providers of healthcare in America, as well as one of the largest providers of sex education. They are in the news a lot because they are often the only providers of abortion services in some areas, but they also provide a full range of healthcare services for men and women. Their website is also a great resource to learn more about anything related to sexual health.

THE NATIONAL DOMESTIC VIOLENCE HOTLINE

www.thehotline.org

The National Domestic Violence Hotline is an emergency phone line (1-800-799-7233) for victims of domestic violence, providing immediate assistance to anyone who needs it.

RAINN

www.rainn.org

The Rape, Abuse & Incest National Network also operates a sexual assault help line (1-800-656-4673), and they run programs for survivors of sexual and domestic abuse.